MW01167093

Making Life Better
Helps Takes the Sting out of
Life with Acid Reflux

" . . . full of positive energy, easy to read and encouraging. Bound to be of great help."
— *Patricia Winters, Ph.D., R.N., C.S.*

" . . . having worked with thousands of doctors on reflux I can tell you that this book is a must read for any parent with a child who suffers from it."
— *Macarena Rose, Inventor of the Prop up Pillow (for acid reflux) http://www.propuppillow.com*

"When a baby has reflux the whole family can suffer. Inside are great common sense suggestions to reduce the stress . . . and help things get better."
— *Edward Freeman, MD, Killeen, TX*

"This book is full of survival tips for stressed–out parents."
— *Jan Burns, Associate Director, PAGER*

"I only wish I had the opportunity to read this book when my daughter was born with reflux."
— *Tamara Gasior, LCSW-C, mother of infant with reflux*

"I wholeheartedly recommend this wonderful book to parents of children suffering from reflux."
— *Marcella Bothwell, MD, University of Missouri*

Making Life Better

for a Baby with Acid Reflux

By

Tracy Davenport, M.A. and
Mike Davenport, Ed.D.

Making Life Better for a Baby with Acid Reflux

ISBN: 0-9639300-x-x

Produced and distributed by SportWork, Inc.
Main Street • P.O. Box 192 • Church Hill, MD • 21623
(410) 556-6030 (phone/fax)
tdavenport2@washcoll.edu
www.makinglifebetter.org

Printed in the United States of America

To an industrial-strength marriage

Table of Contents

FOREWORD

Most important writing is born out of passion and often out of frustration. The authors of this book are passionate about their children and their health. Unfortunately, they have suffered the incredible frustration of watching their second child endure uncontrollable pain almost since birth. Their quest for medical help for their son nearly shattered the very family that they were struggling so hard to save.

In veterinary medicine, we are trained to collect data and to reach diagnoses much as physicians are, but our patients don't speak. Animals' caregivers provide observations that are invaluable in any effective treatment plan.

The Davenports learned (repeatedly) that there are some in the health-care field who are incapable of listening to or comprehending a parent's insight into his own child. And there are others who compassionately devote their careers to the smallest human patients. These patients are often the most difficult to manage correctly.

Hopefully upon reading this book you will be a better advocate for your family in whatever crisis has led you here. You will be empowered to find only the best professionals for your child's treatment and you will know that there are many others who have struggled along the same road before you.

Thanks to caring professionals, to ongoing research, and to your own persistence, improving your and your child's quality of life may be only a phone call or a mouse click away.

Kim Fincher Clabaugh
Doctor of Veterinary Medicine
Chestertown, Maryland
December 2003

The Beginning

It's 4:10 am. We've been wide awake with a screaming four-month-old infant for two hours. He awoke crying, drank half of his bottle, arched his back, and then the real screaming started.

The poor fellow is pulling his ears. He is thrashing out of control and jamming his fingers into his mouth. He is pulling our hair. It's hard to believe that a baby so small could cry so loud, for so long.

But we're not angry—we know that his pain has got to be terrible.

And so begins another typical day in the life with our son who has acid reflux.

The term *colic* may soon be officially a thing of the past and *acid reflux* may take its place. *Reflux*, as it is more commonly called, occurs when the valve in a person's esophagus does not close, or does not stay closed properly, allowing the stomach contents to escape. This valve, the lower esophageal sphincter (LES) works well in most infants; however, current estimates are that upwards of 20% of babies spit up (which is a nonmedical reflux) and about 5–8% of them have other symptoms (which makes it a medical problem). When reflux occurs and the contents escape they can burn the delicate lining of the esophagus, causing pain and damage. Signs and symptoms of reflux may include irritability, sudden or constant crying, food refusal, sleeplessness, and frequent infections. A few babies even have reflux "disease" (a.k.a. GERD), which means that the reflux has caused damage or other serious health consequences.

Unfortunately, our son is in that special percentage whose valve does not work properly. Starting in the second week of his life it became apparent that something was wrong—very wrong. And since that moment, our lives have been very different.

In the pages that follow is the story of how our family copes with acid reflux. It is what we do to survive as best we can, and to help our son. It is also what we wish we would have done sooner. We hope that some of this information may help you.

We also hope that not another baby or family has to suffer through what ours has endured.

What the Heck Is Going On?

Flashback to 1996.

Our first child is born. All is well. The child and mom are healthy. The baby does his part and does baby-type stuff. We do our part and do parent-type stuff. We clothe, bathe, and care for him, and we cruise along without a concern in the world.

No problem. Things are great. He plays and develops and in all essence is your normal, healthy baby.

Then six years later our second child is born. And is our world rocked.

He is healthy—for two weeks. Our only hint of impending trouble is that he will only sleep in his car seat, and he refuses to sleep in his crib. Then things change quickly. He hardly ever eats. And when he does he is either screaming, or vomiting, or both. He rarely sleeps, and when he is awake there are hours and hours and hours of crying.

He tries to do baby-type stuff and we try to do parent-type
stuff like we did with our first child—but no way. Instead,
there are doctors and hospitals and tests and pain and waiting
and more tests and medications. Lots of medications. The
child had taken more medications in his short life than we
have in all our years.

And there is doubt, anxiety, fear, and most of all uncertainty.
Uncertainty that we are good parents. Uncertainty that we
know what the heck we are doing. That uncertainty is fueled
by the lack of a definite answer that we just didn't receive
from the medical community. And one question keeps circling
in our mind: "What the heck is going on?"

We are pushed, we are stretched, and we are stressed like we
had never been before. Our family is damn lucky to survive.

The Dark Side

When Benjamin, our second son, got sick, we did what most
parents do: we responded to the call for help. Our goal was to
get him better, and so we did everything that we could. We
went to doctors, tried new formulas, and recorded sleep patterns. We read and researched.

You name it, we tried it.

There were hours and hours of screaming per day (sometimes
up to six hours per day), and sleepless nights. Our child was in
pain. All of that slowly but surely ate away at our ability to
communicate, our ability to help, our ability to function. We
ended up being pushed—pushed right to the brink of sanity.
Right up to the edge.

A little more pushing and who knows, our marriage and family may not have survived.

If you're a parent you most likely know what we're talking about. Under stress and sleep deprivation it is very easy to lose your ability to communicate clearly and to be non-emotional. And when that happens, families suffer.

For years we tried to conceive Benjamin. Along the way there were several heart-wrenching miscarriages, but we kept trying, despite what could have been further heartache. And now can you imagine that just four months into his life there were times when we said, "What have we done here?"

And we weren't the only ones to feel that way. No one was overly excited about spending time with Benjamin because time with him was really intensive parenting time. There was very little "goo-goo" or warm cuddly time. It was very hard and physically draining, and mentally very difficult. For when you had Benjamin you literally couldn't put him down, and there was little that could be done to console him.

How hard it was became apparent one weekend when we visited Lori, Benjamin's aunt. Benjamin was six months old and had been having a very tough time. Lori, knowing we needed a break, asked us to come visit her in New York City. She babysat Benjamin while we went right next door to a see a movie. This was one of the first times we had been out since Benjamin was born. We were gone exactly one hour and 43 minutes (we know; we timed it). When we returned from the theater and the elevator doors opened on Lori's floor, we could hear Ben's wailing from the other end of the hall. As we ran to Lori's apartment and burst in, Benjamin was in Lori's arms and both were crying. Here were two humans, who had spent the last 60 or more minutes crying because Benjamin's stomach hurt him. They didn't visit; they didn't play like an aunt and nephew should. All they could do was survive.

It was at that point that she and we knew things were out of control and we had to look—really look—for help. We looked for articles, for books, for any resource we could find. Like any educated parent in similar circumstances, we scoured the Web. And we found stuff, like a wonderful support group called Pediatric Adolescent Gastroesophageal Reflux Association (PAGER) who has a very helpful Web site at http://www.reflux.org, and that has had a major impact on our collective lives. Yet, we could not locate much in terms of practical guides to help parents and families in similar circumstances as ours. That's when we decided to write this book.

This Book

With that said, let us tell you a little bit about this book. Our goal is not to relate horror stories or tales meant to keep you up all night (that is, if you are sleeping at all).

Instead, the goal we are striving for is to have this book be a guide to help you. Based on our experiences and the knowledge we have gained along the way, we hope to offer you suggestions, recommendations, and resource avenues to help you get through what Dr. Bill Sears has called a time that "is going to be tough. It may be one of the toughest things you have ever done."[i]

What's Inside

We are both very straightforward people, and with that in mind, we would like to start that type of relationship with you right now.

This book is about how a family survived (and continues to survive) an infant diagnosed with gastroesphogeal reflux (GER) and gastroesphogeal reflux disease (GERD). It is about what we do (and did) to help our child and to help our family survive through some very difficult and trying times. It is also about what we wished we would have done differently and what we know now that we wish we would have known then. Through this, we hope to be able to help you and your family improve the quality of your life.

The advice we offer is specific for the parents, family, and relatives of a baby with acid reflux and it is designed to do one thing, and one thing only—to help those folks survive the hardship that goes hand in hand with a child with this affliction. To help you, we have divided this information into ten steps.

Prior to having a sick child, we would have easily dismissed many of the horror stories that abound about living with an infant with acid reflux. Now that we have a child diagnosed with it (and still suffering from it) we don't dismiss a single story. In fact, we tend to think that most of those stories grossly underestimate the toll that is taken on the child's, parents', family's, and relatives' quality of life.

What's Not Inside

There are some good folks who are working long and hard trying to solve the mystery of infant acid reflux, and they are trying to develop solutions for those who suffer from it. There are a few resources where you can get sound advice about the medical problem. If it is medical advice you need please turn to your family physician, pediatrician, or other professional health-care provider. We want you to know that you will not find medical advice, medical recommendations, or diagnostic assistance here.

Medical advice offered by lay people can be very counterproductive and possibly even dangerous. If it is medical assistance you need to care for your child, make sure that you contact a qualified medical professional. For suggestions about finding capable medical assistance, see Steps 3 and 4 in the upcoming chapters.

---

[i] Reflux Digest. (Summer, 2002. V 6, N 1). Interview with Bill Sears, MD. p. 4.

Ten Steps to Improving the Quality of Life When Your Baby Has Acid Reflux

We want to say this right up front: In the course of Benjamin's illness and subsequent treatments we have met some wonderful, caring, hardworking, and amazing people. We have met professionals who have tried and tried and tried to help us and Benjamin. (Unfortunately, we've also met folks who were not so helpful and some who were actually harmful . . . but that is another story for another book.)

At the time we came face to face with it, acid reflux was just beginning to be truly understood and diagnosed. This disorder, gastroesphogeal reflux, or "GER" as it is more commonly known, is, in very simple mechanical terms, a plumbing problem with the digestive system. Although that may sound simple, this disease can be anything but and can turn into a very complex illness that can cause multiple problems, can be tricky to diagnose, and problematic to treat if the physician is not experienced with reflux. And this disease, as one pediatrician we know put it, can be *horrific*. And he was right—very right.

THE TEN STEPS

There are ten specific things (we call them *Steps*) that we have done during the course of Benjamin's illness that have had a major positive impact on his and our family's quality of life.

Before we get into details, let us tell you two things about these ten steps. First, some of them saved Benjamin, our marriage, and our family. No exaggeration there—they literally saved us in a time of crisis.

Second, some of these steps might not work for you—although we hope that many or all of them will. However, that's not important. What is really important is that you realize that having a baby with reflux can be terribly intensive and that you will need to be very involved and possibly take steps that you might not typically take with a healthy child to get through the tough times ahead. (If these steps don't work for you, our hope is that you might try them again later, or that they might prompt you to discover other steps that will work.)

Following is a list of the ten steps that we discuss in this book:

1) Understand How Dang Hard This Might Be
2) Remember that the Baby Isn't Bad; the Pain Is!
3) Take Charge
4) Be Sure They Are Working for You
5) Research It to the Bone
6) Build Support
7) Recharge Your Batteries
8) Stay Healthy
9) Be Prepared to Spend Money
10) Know that It's Not Over Until It's Over

How to Get the Most from This Book

By now you should have a fairly good idea what this book is about and about some of the information included. The layout of this book has been arranged to be used as a reference guide. Basically the chapters are arranged in a specific order. As you go through each chapter you will see that they build on the chapter before them—a cumulative effect. But at the same time, if you have a problem with one specific area, you will be able to turn directly to that section for help. If you have a problem and don't know where to turn, flip to the index in the back; we've tried to make it as thorough as possible.

In several of the chapters there are sections entitled *How to Get the Most from This Step*. These are tasks designed to help you get the most from the step. These sections are based on our experiences, our expertise, and suggestions of experts and lay-people in the field. In an attempt to make these sections as accurate as possible, we've had several friends test them (at least they were friends when we started).

<u>Step 1</u>

Understand How Dang Hard This Might Be

Ef you have a baby with acid reflux you might be about to embark on a journey that could be more intense than anything that you have ever done before. Here is why.

Why Will This Be Hard?

We as humans are not hardwired to watch a child, especially an infant, be in pain. When we see an infant suffering we are driven to respond. Our mind and body gear up to do whatever we need to do to help. An infant in pain makes a connection with our very soul. We are motivated. We are pushed. We *must* help.

When that child is our own, the response is raised to an entirely new level of intensity. And therein lies the problem with having a baby with reflux or GERD. You see, the affliction may go away quickly; however, it may last quite a while—and even a few weeks of caring for a baby with reflux can change you forever.

Marian Sandmaier wrote a very poignant article recently for the *Washington Post* in which she describes the intensity of the help-response:

> There comes a moment in a parent's life when you understand that raising a child is less an act of love and fortitude than something much wilder, something that sniffs the wind and bares its fangs at intruders, implacable in its drive to keep its offspring safe. You may not know you have this beast in you; you may see yourself as essentially rational and peaceable, willing to abide by the rules. Then everything changes.[ii]

This drive to protect, to care for a little one who cannot speak and care for himself, can cause stress—a lot of stress. One of the reasons is because normal efforts to comfort usually don't work well with a baby with reflux who is in pain. Over a long time, this stress can mean trouble.

Elevated levels of stress over time can be very destructive. This stress can lead to the phenomenon we commonly know as burnout. Christina Maslach, a noted researcher in burnout and its effects describes burnout as:

> a psychological syndrome of emotional exhaustion, depersonalization of others, and reduced personal accomplishment that can occur among individuals in response to the chronic emotional strain of dealing with other human beings, especially troubled ones.[iii]

A parent who suffers burnout can become emotionally exhausted, non-caring, and feel like he or she is doing a terrible job. And those feelings unabated can turn into trouble. "Children with reflux do try the patience of a saint," says Beth Anderson, Executive Director of PAGER. "Almost all parents we talk to say this is the most stressful experience of their lives and an alarming number admit to fantasies of throwing the baby out the window."[iv]

For a parent of a reflux baby:

- ❖ Your health (mental and physical) may suffer
- ❖ Your family life may suffer
- ❖ Your job may suffer
- ❖ Your baby's health may suffer
- ❖ Your social life may suffer

Your Health May Suffer

Interestingly enough, when Benjamin became sick we were constantly worried about his health—and in turn ours suffered. We have always been pretty healthy folks (we are knocking on wood very hard as we write this) but, boy, did we get rocked. For instance, during one two-week-period, when Benjamin was very sick, one of us came down with a severe case of bronchitis, the other was flattened with physical exhaustion, and our oldest son came down with croup (and had to be taken to the local emergency room at 2:30 A.M.).

This isn't just a phenomenon limited to our family. There are several studies that investigated the effect that caring for a chronically ill child had on the caregiver's health. Some noted significant changes, and some even reported drastic changes to all family members' health.[v]

Our health really suffered and we believe that it was in large part due to sleep deprivation—it was one of the main problems we had. Now this is not the same type of sleep deprivation that goes along with having a healthy infant in the home, occasionally waking here and there. Oh no! This is different—really different. It is sleep deprivation raised to a new level.

There were times when we were getting up every 19 minutes to tend to Benjamin. That in itself was difficult, but then when up, he was not consoled as a normal baby might be. He was up for hours screaming in pain and more often than not it woke the whole house.

One recommendation we received was to have one of us sleep in another part of the house, so as to get a good night's sleep. Unfortunately, this didn't work because when Benjamin awoke it was with a cry oftentimes so terribly horrific that it could (and probably more than once did) wake the whole neighborhood.

Besides the sleep issue, our backs paid a price. Why? Because this was a baby who could not be put down; he had to be constantly held in an upright position just to relieve his pain and give him emotional support.

What accentuated the toll on our health was that the onset of reflux was so slow and that the diagnosis was difficult to attain. We cannot speak for others but with Benjamin, when he was born, we were (as most parents are) somewhat braced to hear the news that something might be wrong. After several days, when everything seemed normal, we happily exhaled. However, after two weeks the reflux began to appear, when we had already taken for granted that our baby was healthy, and by that time our support team had left the job (assuming that all was well).

And it took us quite a while to get a diagnosis of reflux—it took several months, in fact.

Your Finances May Suffer

Having a child with reflux can create a great financial burden. For instance, it was almost impossible for one of us to run off to work and leave our partner alone caring for both Benjamin and our other son. When we tried to work at home, there was no longer any peaceful space available. So we had to hire a lot of babysitters to help.

We also found that we needed extra help just to do the simple little things that we normally did before Benjamin, stuff like cleaning the house, going grocery shopping, or doing yard work. With a healthy baby, things go on, just at a much slower pace. With a reflux baby, everything can come to a screeching halt, and to get back on track you might need to spend money.

We also found that a lack of organization crept into our life with our high-needs baby. When our life got turned upside down this played havoc on our financial situation. For the first time in a 16-year marriage we missed mortgage and car insurance payments, and bounced checks.

And then there were the doctor's bills. Benjamin was at a doctor's appointment or a hospital practically every week of his life for the first six months. At one point, he was taking medication nine times per day. Even the small co-pay was adding up, not to mention the medicines that he was on and that he drank a formula that cost over $60 a week.

And last, but by no means least, is the possibility of legal bills. While many folks won't encounter legal troubles with a reflux baby it is a sad state of affairs today that some of you will. We offer tips and suggestions about your finances in *Step 9: Be Prepared to Spend Money.*

Your Mental State May Suffer

We've got to tell you, your mental state may very well be at risk when dealing with a reflux baby. The disrupted social life, personal strain, economic uncertainty, and insecurity about the baby's health can all add up to a high level of stress.[vi] And that is what happened to us—we got worn down by the unremitting elevated level of stress.

Well . . . worn down isn't quite strong enough—more like crushed.

Testifying before Congress, Jan Burns, Assistant Director of PAGER, related her own experience about her child with reflux:

> I had successfully raised two other children and had a Master's degree in early intervention with 13 years of experience, but even a medical degree couldn't have prepared me for the sleep

> deprivation and the 24/7 intensive care parenting required to care for such a critically ill child.[vii]

Caring for a baby with reflux can be crushing. Here is an analogy: When the body goes into shock due to blood loss, it attempts to protect the brain from damage due to lack of blood. The body begins to shut down parts that are not absolutely critical to its survival. For example, one of the first body parts to go is the stomach. The brain shuts it down, and sends the blood elsewhere (that is why one of the first signs of shock is nausea and vomiting).

What happened to us was very much like this compensation for shock. It was like our brains were trying to protect themselves from the overload of stress, and so the non-priority items were dropped. For instance, we rarely went out to eat or to a movie, two things we enjoyed pre-Ben.

Unfortunately, some of the other things that helped us compensate for the stress were dropped—like exercise—and that made the stress cycle build on itself.

Another thing that went was the yard and house upkeep. We just didn't have the time and energy to do the yard work and clean the house. And each time we came home and looked around, there was a constant reminder of how difficult things actually were, and of course that generated more stress.

Then, there was the strain of the unknown, and this came in three flavors. First, there was the pressure of not knowing what was wrong with Benjamin. Second, there was the pressure of not knowing for sure when he was going to get better.

(People told us it would be over in 3 months, then in 6 months. With Ben, just when it felt like things were getting better, he took a turn for the worse. It took another month and many doctors' appointments and diagnostic procedures to find out that Benjamin had a yeast infection, followed by a reaction to a reflux medication.) Third, there was the pressure of not knowing exactly what to do to comfort Benjamin.

For our thoughts on how to reduce the negative impact to your mental health, turn to *Step 7: Recharge Your Batteries*.

Your Family May Suffer

A reflux baby's suffering can significantly impact the quality of life for an entire family. It seems pretty reasonable to suggest that a crisis affecting one family member will affect all other family members.[viii]

One of our saddest moments happened when we had directed our oldest son, Brook, to play on his own while we cared for the baby. He did something quite special while playing and he hurriedly came to report on his accomplishment, but we couldn't even hear him over Benjamin's screaming. This just added to our guilt and feelings of inadequacy, not only as parents to the baby, but now we were losing our confidence with our oldest as well.

Additionally, where days off from work were once filled with outings that included everyone, things were changed because one parent had to stay with Ben, so there was rarely a time when everyone was together.

Overall, we were just less excited about life—we were usually pretty good first thing in the morning, but when things were at their worst, we even awoke feeling defeated.

Your Job May Suffer

There has been some very interesting research done on the effects of stress in the workplace, and how that stress spills over to home life. One thing that was found was that the stress of work often came home with the worker, and does not stay at work.[ix]

The same is true in the other direction—the stress of home rarely stays just there; instead, it often travels to work. And that spillover to work can be very noticeable and very destructive.

When we were at work it was pretty noticeable that often we were just there physically, and not mentally. And sometimes, hardly even there physically.

Your Social Life May Suffer

Almost without saying, having a baby changes your social life. This phenomenon becomes really apparent with a reflux baby, because going out with a reflux baby can often be too unpredictable. Things can get wild and crazy and can spiral out of control without warning.

One thing that we discovered was that it was extremely difficult to go out and leave Benjamin at home, because it was often too darn hard to find a sitter who could care for him. On the few times that we did go out we would call only to hear an exasperated sitter on the line with a screaming baby in the background, and we quickly found ourselves on the way home.

Two months into this, already weary and exhausted beyond our imaginations, we decided to give ourselves a break and go out and get a bite to eat. To do this we had to hire two baby-sitters: one for our oldest son, Brook, and one for Benjamin. Brook was very excited since we hired his favorite sitter to play with him. We were gone about an hour and on returning we found Benjamin having such a difficult time that both sitters were with him (probably in large part to give each other moral support) and poor Brook just ended up playing by himself the entire time.

Realize this—finding a sitter for a healthy child can be hard, but finding one to watch a child with GER can be downright impossible.

And how about taking the child with you? Well, Sharmi Banik, a writer for the *Germantown Gazette,* describes an interesting aspect of a social life with an infant suffering with GERD:

> Imagine a casual trip to Lakeforest Mall with your baby, when suddenly he starts to scream, shake, turn blue and then projectile vomits on a well-dressed woman more than five feet away.[x]

As you might imagine, all this can put a major crimp in any social life.

HOW TO GET THE MOST FROM THIS STEP

How Hard Is It?

Problem: Your baby suffers from reflux and you want to get an idea of how difficult things are—great information to know in order to evaluate where you might need help.

Needed: Form 1, pencil/pen, about fifteen minutes.

Before we begin, a few words of caution here: First, while your feelings of stress and strain may be very real, you should be cautious about whom you express them to. A pediatrician's main goal is the care of a child, and not necessarily you—an adult. This means that the pediatrician's office may not be a safe environment to express feelings of stress and strain. (However, keep in mind that each doctor is different.) You might find a safer environment with your own doctor, a medical therapist, or a support group such as PAGER (http://www.reflux.org).

Step 1: Concentrate. Find some quiet time and then flip to the two-page assessment form.

Step 2: Complete the form. Answer each step to the best of your ability. You might want to consider having you and your partner complete this form separately, and then compare scores.

Step 3: Take a break. When complete, put the form down for a period of time (usually a day or two) and then review it.

Step 4: Complete the form and score it. Take your score and compare it to the scale at the end of the form. From there, follow the recommendations, or consider taking action that may be appropriate for you based on the results.

FORM 1: HOW HARD IS IT?

Step 1: You're trying to get an idea of how intense caring for your high-needs baby is. Answer the following questions by filling in the blank with one of these responses that best describes your state of mind.

Excellent	*Very Good*	*Good*	*Poor*	*Terrible*
5pts	4pts	3pts	2pts	1pt

Score	Questions
1. _____	I feel that I am a(n) _____ influence on my family
2. _____	I am doing a(n) _____ job of caring for my baby.
3. _____	My relationship with my significant other is _____ .
4. _____	Compared to pre-baby, my house/apartment is in _____ condition.
5. _____	My relationships with my best friends are _____ compared to pre-baby.
6. _____	At the end of the day, my emotional state is _____ .

Form 1 continues next page

35

Form 1, continued

7. _____   I am doing a(n) _____ job at my
              work.

8. _____   In the morning, I feel _____ .

9. _____   Being with my baby is _____ for
              me.

Total score: _____

Step 2: Scoring. Now go back to each question. In the left-hand column you gave yourself the following points:

For each answer of	Give yourself
Excellent	5 points
Very good	4 points
Good	3 points
Poor	2 points
Terrible	1 points

Step 3: Total it up. Now take your total score and compare it to the following chart. This will give you an idea of what action you might want to take. Keep in mind that the following are only recommendations based on common sense, and not specifically on medical guidance.

If you score is in this range	You might want to consider doing this:
40 to 45 points	You're doing great. Congratulate yourself!
30 to 39 points	Take special care of yourself and family members so that things don't get any worse. Refer to Step 8 for suggestions.
20 to 29 points	Get support from family, friends, and PAGER. Refer to Step 6 for suggestions.
9 to 19 points	Talk to your general practitioner or a medical illness therapist since you might need an ally in convincing the doctors that your child is suffering.*

* Because your child's doctor is only responsible for your child, he may not be the best person with whom to discuss your stress.

[ii] Sandmaier, M. (2003). Listening for zebras. Washingtonpost.com. PHE01.

[iii] Maslach, C. (1993). Burnout: A multidimensional perspective. In W. B. Schaufeli, C. Maslach, & T. Marek (Eds.), Professional burnout: Recent developments in theory and research (pp. 19-32). Washington D.C.: Taylor & Francis.

[iv] Bundle of misery. (August 27, 2002). The Washington Post, p. F6.

[v] Tomlinson, P.S., Kotchevar, J., & Swanson, L. (1995). Caregiver mental health and family health outcomes following critical hospitalization of a child. Issues in Mental Health Nursing, 16, 533

[vi] Patterson, J. M., Leonard, B., & Titus, J. C. (1992). Home care for medically fragile children: impact on family health and well-being. Development and Behavioral Pediatrics, 13, 4.

[vii] Reflux Digest. (June 2003, V7, N2). PAGER testifies before Congress. p. 1.

[viii] Patterson, J. M., Leonard, B., & Titus, J. C. (1992). Home care for medically fragile children: impact on family health and well-being. Development and Behavioral Pediatrics, 13, 4.

[ix] Leiter, M. P., & Durup, J. M. (1996). Work, home, and in-between: A longitudinal study of spillover. Journal of Applied Behavioral Science, 31 (1), 29-47.

[x] Banik, S. Childhood heartburn disease causes parent's grief. (1994, May 18). Germantown Gazette, A1.

Step 2

Remember that the Baby Isn't Bad; the Pain Is!

If you find yourself reading this book, especially reading this chapter, more than likely, you are sleep deprived, your life/work schedule is in chaos, your child is possibly facing medical treatment, and/or you do not yet have a successful course of treatment. All of the above can contribute to reducing your patience with your crying baby.

Parents of a healthy baby are usually asked to tend to a crying baby every so often. For them, it is easy to respond with infinite patience, caring words, and great empathy. However, parents of a baby with GER are asked to respond to a baby in discomfort almost continuously. Additionally, common methods of comforting the baby usually don't work, and this can be more than discouraging. Because of this, it is sometimes difficult to remember that it is not the baby that is bad, but it is the baby's pain that is bad.

And this is compounded when the reflux is not diagnosed promptly or properly. When Benjamin's symptoms first appeared we were told everything under the sun to explain his intense crying—from it was the "mom's fault," to he was just "precocious," to he was just trying to get attention. It became apparent that either we were not explaining his symptoms well enough or his pain was not being taken seriously. When we finally did get good care we found out that our child's reflux was severely abnormal and that his esophagus was getting an acid bath over 150 times a day!

If a physician is not experienced with reflux then he or she may become impatient with there not being a quick fix. Unfortunately, this can lead to frustration and blame. This happens more than it should with infant reflux. Here is one such story related in *Reflux Digest*:

> Our son . . . suffered with reflux from birth. He was 15 months of age before I found anyone who would really believe just how much pain he almost constantly endured. He woke crying in very real pain anywhere from 8 to 14 times each and every night.[xi]

We've talked to dozens upon dozens of adults who have acid reflux. It absolutely floors us the stories they relate about their pain, their discomfort, their altered and disruptive sleep patterns, and what the reflux episodes feel like. Here are adults who are in pain—yet they have an outlet, they can voice their pain in words.

Now for one moment let's assume that your baby has the same pain that these adults have. The baby cannot talk, so she has only one way to voice her pain—and that is by crying. Well, probably not just crying, but instead, gut-wrenching screaming and howling that can go on and on for hours. The baby is communicating with you and what she is telling you is:

> "I AM IN PAIN! It is not my choice, I don't want it to happen, and there is nothing that I can do to stop it. I am a VICTIM here too!"

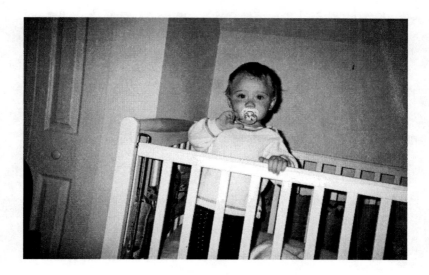

Babies don't have a voice to explain their pain.

It is therefore important that you respond appropriately to the only language the baby has. One way to check in to see if you are is by reviewing the language that you use to describe your baby's situation. For instance, saying that your baby is "fussy," "precocious," or "demanding" suggests that you think that your baby might be making a conscious decision to be in pain or to frequently wake up. That is pretty darn unlikely.

HOW TO GET THE MOST FROM THIS STEP

Are You Blaming the Baby?

Problem: Time to check in to see if you are blaming the baby for his or her misery.

Step 1: Your words are important. A vital step in not blaming the baby for the pain is using words that describe the baby's innocence. Your words are incredibly powerful and often set the tone for your mood and your ability to care for your baby.

Step 2: Listen. Register in your mind which of the following examples of communication do and do not blame the baby for being in pain.

Blaming the Baby	Blaming the Pain
The baby kept me up all night last night.	The baby had a difficult night last night.
The baby wouldn't let me put him down all day.	He really needed me to hold him all day to provide him some relief.
The baby just spit up on my new sweater and ruined it.	The baby wasn't able to keep his last bottle down.
The baby's constant crying is driving me nuts.	The baby seems especially uncomfortable today.

Step 3: Notice any trends? Now listen to your own references to your baby's and family's discomfort and try to be conscious of how you are expressing the situation. Notice any similarities to the choices above?

Your words, your language, can give you insight into how you view your baby's pain, and this is critical. We found that once we could get our arms around the pure agony that Benjamin was going through we were much better able to help him, and in turn improve the quality of his and our life.

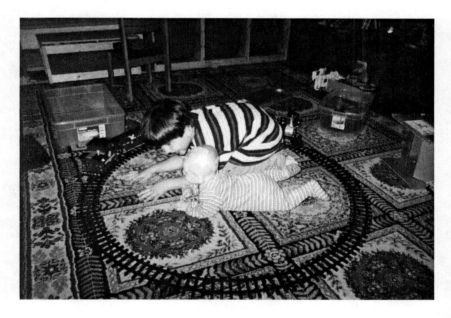

As we began to better manage Benjamin's pain his older brother began to really enjoy having a baby brother.

[xi] Reflux Digest. (Summer 2001. V 5, N 2). [Letter to the editor]. p. 10

<u>Step 3</u>

Take Charge

T his is different—so very different. Caring for a baby suffering from reflux is different in so many respects from caring for a healthy child. Why? Because GER is a complex illness, just now beginning to be somewhat understood, involving patients who in many cases cannot be helpful in treatment because they cannot yet talk, and the emotions can be so high and the discomfort so intense.

Because this is so different—and the stakes so high—you are going to be required to do things differently than you probably ever have had to do them before. And the big difference—you will need to *take charge*.

Take charge? You? Yup.

Here is what we mean by taking charge. There is information that will be needed—*you* will have to get that. There will be appointments that will have to be juggled—that's *your* responsibility. You might have to, want to, or need to travel to get the best care—that's on *your* shoulders. And all the while *you* will have to advocate very hard for your child.

Get Information

At no other time is it more apparent that things are different (and that you will need to take charge) than when you are trying to get information about your child and the illness.

With a typically healthy family, parents talk to other parents about their kids. Hang around a bowling alley and parents are discussing how and what their kids are doing. Go to a mom's group and comparisons are happening all over the place about how kids are sleeping, who's eating what, and how tall kids are. However, because babies with GER require totally different parenting techniques you're not going to hear much information that will be helpful unless there are parents of babies suffering from reflux there. (In fact, talking to parents of healthy children can make you even feel worse.)

For you to find out what is going on with your child and to keep the quality of life as good as possible, you will need to assume responsibility and that means searching for information in non-typical, special places.

Here is an instance: Beth Anderson, the Founding Director of PAGER, began a support group for parents of reflux kids (http://www.reflux.org) to help herself get information about what was going on. Beth took charge, and here is what she wrote in one of her newsletters:

> When the group started, it was predicted that
> we would never find more than ten mothers

whose kids had the "rare" disease. This didn't deter us since the main reason for starting the group was to get advice from other people and learn what to do for our own miserable little "gerdlings." We suspected that we might find a hundred families, but even we had no clue that eventually 10,000 people every month would find us [on our Web site].

A common scenario is that when your child begins to first show signs of reflux you go to your family doctor. If your family doctor needs more information on diagnosing and treating he may send you to a pediatrician. If the pediatrician needs more information, she may send you to a specialist such as a gastroentronologist. If the gastroentronologist needs more information he might send you to an allergist, a respiratory specialist, or an ear, nose, and throat specialist for tests.

The above illustration is one way in which a physician might get more information about a patient's illness. However, it is not nearly as clear-cut for parents of these special babies how they get information. But there are several things that you can do. At the end of this chapter you will find a section to help you get the most of this step. To get further insight into gathering information about reflux, turn to *Step 5: Research It to the Bone.*

Make More Than One Appointment

Appointments, appointments, appointments. Odds are good that there are going to be one heck of a lot of doctors' appointments popping up on your calendar. That means someone needs to be responsible for organizing them, and don't under-estimate how critical this job will be. In one ten-day period we had ten doctors' appointments. That took an enormous amount of juggling between our work schedules, our other son's schedule, and just life as a whole to make it work.

Speaking of appointments, we need to make this specific rec-ommendation:

> *MAKE AN APPOINTMENT FOR TWO DIFFERENT DOCTORS IN TWO DIFFERENT PLACES IF YOU ARE REFERRED TO A SPECIALIST!*

(If you think that when you see something written in all capital letters that person is yelling, well . . . you're correct in this in-stance. We are yelling this recommendation, as loud as the print on this page will let us.)

Here is why you should make two appointments. Getting in with these professionals can take months and months. Believe us, we know that getting in to see any specialist will seem like a relief to you and your family. However, you want to protect yourself in case a referral doesn't work out.

Unfortunately, there are some medical professionals that not only don't know about reflux and GERD, some of them will even "fake it" and dispense bad information and maybe even bad medications or a bad diagnosis. You don't want to have the misfortune of waiting a very long time to get in to see someone like this.

For instance, we were working with a GI nurse at a teaching hospital and were describing to her the terrible sleeping problems that Benjamin was having. Her response was, "I've never heard of reflux keeping anyone awake before." (When we finally did get good help and related that story to another GI nurse at another teaching hospital, her reply was, "What planet was she from?")

It happens occasionally that, when a child isn't thriving and the doctors don't have a firm answer, they start blaming the mother. If you have any inkling that this might be happening to you, grab your diaper bag and run for the door as quickly as you can. And you don't want to have to wait another three months to see someone else.

If you do make two appointments, you can always cancel the second appointment if you sense that the first doctor is right on track with helping your child (more about this in the next chapter).

Hit the Road

Another area you will want to step up and take charge of is your willingness to travel. In the course of Ben's care it was necessary for us to go to five different hospitals in four different states. You may have to travel to get the best care for your child, but it may be well worth it. Too much time with a misdiagnosis just adds to heartache and unnecessary fatigue. Find where the best doctors are and go there. Don't settle for second best just because it is closer to home. We did one time and it almost destroyed our family.

Another reason to travel is that different places may use different technology in diagnosis and treatment of reflux. The next two figures show two different types of pH probes that were used on Benjamin to diagnose the severity of his reflux. In one test we had to stay in a hospital setting while the test was conducted. The other photo shows a remote sensing pH probe that allowed us to leave the hospital during the test. As you can see there is a happy boy in only one picture.

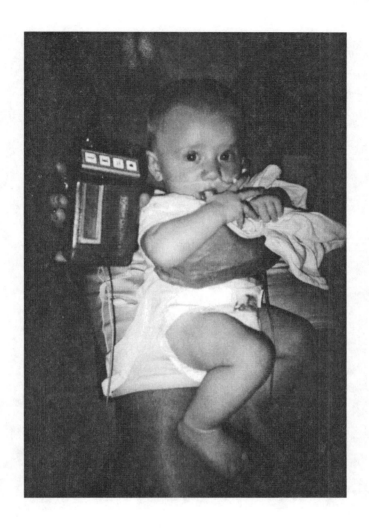

Conventional two-channel pH probe

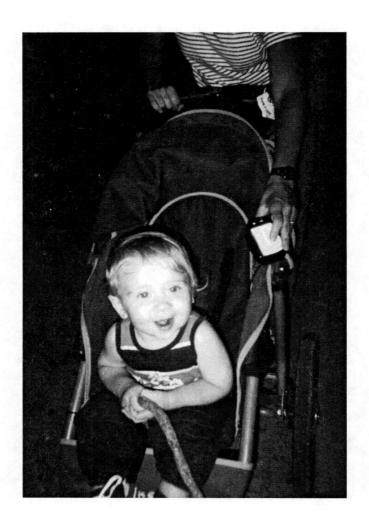

Remote sensing pH probe at
University of Missouri-Columbia

And, yes, this will cost money, but your baby's health and quality of life may well depend on it. In the end you may well save money by getting the best medical care as soon as possible. See *Step 9: Be Prepared to Spend Money* for more about the costs you might incur.

Push Hard

Your baby is crying for a reason. As parents you want and need to know why. To do that, you might have to push hard to find out what is wrong. What we mean is that you might well need to be assertive and strong willed to get to the bottom of the problem.

Your child is ill. Every time he screams, he is saying, "HELP ME!" He needs an advocate, someone to campaign for him, to find out what is wrong and to fix it.

You'll need to trust your instincts here. We guarantee you that the moment your child is no longer in pain, you will ask yourself if you did everything in your power to make things better for him as quickly as you could.

Caution

Be cautious. If someone says, "I don't know," as an answer to a question about your baby's health, then your follow up question should be, "How do we find out the answer?"

Anyone worth their salt will want to get the baby better as much as you do, and will be willing to work hard to get there. If you do not sense that this is the case, either you are not presenting the case in a mature way, or the caregiver doesn't realize the severity of the situation. If at ANY time, you feel that a medical professional may be looking for a way out of what might be a very difficult and frustrating situation by blaming you, immediately RUN, don't walk, for the door.

HOW TO GET THE MOST FROM THIS STEP

Gathering Data About Your Child's Reflux

Problem: You are in charge and you need to track important information.

Knowledge is power, and that saying is so truthful when it comes to the signs of your child's reflux. (A *sign* is an observed indication of an illness, as compared to a *symptom*, which is an indication felt by the patient.) The more you know about the signs, the better care you can give to your child and get for your child. This task is designed to help you gather some objective knowledge in what is probably a very emotional and difficult time. The steps are simple, but don't underestimate how powerful this information can be.

For us, knowing the signs made a critical difference in Benjamin's care. He was exhibiting many of the classic signs of reflux (arching, screaming, food refusal, multiple awakenings, vomiting). Once we started tracing those signs, patterns became apparent. From that information we learned that certain foods seemed to increase the signs. We also noticed that different positions (holding, sleeping) made a difference in the number and severity of signs. And we began to see that some of the medications prescribed for Benjamin actually were making him sicker.

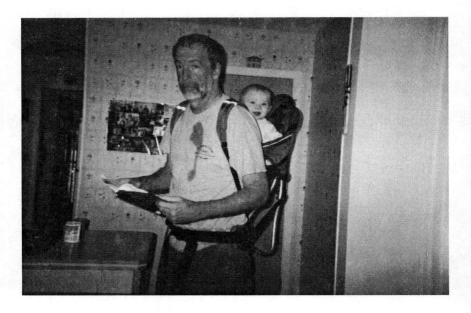

Benjamin seemed to do best in an upright position. However, before we could get him in the backpack he refluxed on his dad.

Knowledge is power, and you need knowledge because you are in charge. In most cases the doctors will only see your child for a small window of time, and doctors have running through their head massive amounts of published biological and medical literature, and are usually extremely busy. You are the ones who are observing your child day and night.

Step 1: Prepare to track. You need to track your child's signs, so get ready. You'll need a tracking sheet, writing utensil, and a plan for tracking.

Step 2: Get a form. We've included a sample form we made to track Benjamin's signs. If you want to copy it directly from this book, you can, you just might need to set the copier to an enlarged size to make the copy more user friendly. We use (we often still track) one form per day. If you want to make your own form, try this . . .

Step 3: Do it yourself. If you are computer literate, and you have Excel or any other spreadsheet program, it should take you about 10 minutes to make a tracking-form template. The most difficult part for us was to figure out exactly what items we wanted to track. This took about two weeks of trial and error, and as you can see on our form, we really got down to the basics.

We suggest that you include a 24-hour axis, so that you can note when the signs occurred. Additionally, we recommend that you note the exact time when you give medications. This step is important for two reasons. First, you might see patterns emerge related to the medications and the signs. Second, you really need to know when you give medications.

This can be critical because some medications need to be given at a specific amount of time before meals and some at a specific amount of time after meals. But that really is secondary to the fact that if your child is ill enough to be on medication you are probably sleep deprived or at least just distracted. If you are, you need to take steps to ensure you are giving the proper dosage. This is really important when more than one person might be giving the medications.

Step 4: Collect and copy. When you start accumulating forms, make a copy of them for your own records, and store them away in a safe place. Then, at your next doctor's appointment, take the originals in and discuss them with your health-care team. Especially note to them any trends you've noticed.

To assist you in taking charge, the following form will give you a format in which to record information and observations to present to your health-care provider in an objective manner.

TIME →	3A	4A	5A	6A	7A	8A	9A	10A	11A	12P	1P	2P	3P	4P	5P	6P	7P	8P	9P	10P	11P	12A	1A	2A
SLEEP																								
VOMITING																								
MEDS #1																								
ARCHING																								
MEDS #2																								
PAIN EPISODE																								
CHOKING																								
SNEEZING																								
FOOD																								

Making Life Better —

Step 4

Be Sure They Are Working for You

Here it comes. It's time for a conversation that we've been holding off until now, just to make sure that you're ready for it. It's a big one—a really important one. What we need to tell you is not only one of the most critical concepts in this book, it might well be the most significant working idea that you have while your child is sick. It is, in essence, the birds-and-bees talk for parents of reflux children. What we are about to tell you is going to have a great impact on you, your child, and on your family.

However, before you read any further, do this. Find a quiet place where you can be undisturbed for ten minutes. Go there, turn off the cell phone, pager, fax machine, regular phone, or what have you. Have someone watch the kid(s), sit down and read these words that follow with an open mind. Then reread it in a few days. It is also important to have all family members read it.

Catch This

The medical community works for you and your family!

Seriously, the medical community works for YOU!

It absolutely amazes us how this very simple concept has become so convoluted. Some patients are under the impression that they are at the beck and call of their physicians, that they should blindly go along, unquestioningly, with a doctor's orders, for no other reason than because, well . . . because they are ordered by a doctor. We are here to tell you—not quite. Especially for families of infants and children with acid reflux.

When you hire health-care professionals, you are selecting a medical team to help you get your child better. To use a sports analogy, you are the owner of a sports team, and your primary doctor is the coach. He or she will call the plays; yet in the end, you will have the final say.

Here is one instance we experienced in which the doctor forgot who was the client (who was working for whom). We had just taken Benjamin to the hospital for an evaluation, and in preparing for the visit we read as much as we could find on GER and the medications Benjamin was taking. During the visit, the physician at the hospital came in to look at Benjamin and we began to ask him questions. You could tell he was put off by our questions, which were simple and politely put. Finally, in frustration he looked at us and told us, "Stop reading so much. Leave it to us!"

In essence he told us to shut up and do as we are told. What would you do if you took your car to a mechanic, and he came back and told you that you had this major problem. You then begin to ask him a few questions and he tells you to "just do as I say and stop asking questions!"

New mechanic? You betcha.

You are the boss!!!

Now there are several things that you can do to insure that your relationship with your medical team stays positive and productive, and we are going to discuss those in a moment. But the absolute most important thing you can do, without any doubt, is to keep in mind that . . . *you are the boss, and they are working for you!*

Did you catch that? You are the boss and you have the final say. However, as in the workplace, being the boss is both an inherent privilege and a huge responsibility, and that is no different for the parents of a child with reflux.

How to Be a Great Boss

Okay, so you're the boss. So what are you to do? Well, you need to be the best boss possible because your baby's health is on the line. And being a great boss usually means being a great leader. Now you may not feel like being a leader, especially if you're very tired and worried about your child . . . but you're going to need to be one to get the best care.

Following is a list that can help in your quest. We present these to you to get you thinking in the right direction. For further help in compiling your medical team turn to the end of this chapter.

Hire the best. Part of being a great boss is to make sure you hire the best people available. That makes sense, doesn't it? The best people will do the best work, so why not have them on your team? It seems to us that often patients aren't overly selective about their health-care providers.

Time and again, during our research, we found testimony from parents of infants with reflux who were having a difficult (or impossible) time with their doctors. Now, we know that there are many, many good doctors out there, working long and hard to help, like in this example:

> from the moment I entered the specialist's room on that day, this story took a significant turn from [my other child]. Not only was I believed, but I was asked my opinion, and we discussed the possible causes, treatments, and options open to me, and then he simply asked what I wanted him to do and we discussed it. At all times, I was the one that was given the choice of what was to be done and the direction in which we should head. I came out of that room feeling informed, in charge of the situation, and thus empowered to handle it.[xii]

However, there are also some doctors working in the field, who, like the following example, can make things so much more difficult than they need to be:

> On the fourth day, my Maternal & Child Health Nurse visited. "You need to relax." Lucas (the baby) continued to scream. On the fifth day, the

visiting nurse told me that all babies cried! "But he is screaming," I protested. "There's something wrong." "You're doing fine," she said. On the sixth day, I went to my doctor, "All babies cry," he said. "Try to get some sleep." When I protested that Lucas only slept in 30-minute cycles and only 7 of them in 24 hours, he said, "That is normal, it will get better." It didn't![xiii]

Yes, yes, yes . . . sometimes there is little or no choice at all of providers, due to restrictions such as locality or insurance membership. Yet time and time again we hear of patients who have choices yet go to a questionable doctor for the simple reason of, well . . . "just because."

To insure that you're hiring the best, check the credentials of the doctor(s) that you are going to work with. It is not so important that you ask where they went to medical school, or where they did their residency, but it is really important that you find out about their experience with reflux in infants and with GERD. Find out if there are one or more current patients you could talk to for a reference (this may be difficult due to patient confidentiality issues, but PAGER might be able to help). Ask people whose opinion you hold in high regard whom they might recommend. Do some homework, and then hire the best that you can.

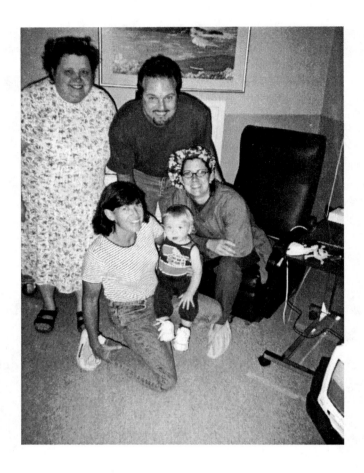

Part of Benjamin's wonderful health-care team at the University of Missouri consists of an advanced nurse, a doctor of pharmacology and an ENT surgeon (pictured left to right).

Blend information. Sometimes you will know things the experts don't. With Benjamin, since we were with him 24/7 we knew his sleeping and eating patterns, we knew what his different cries meant, and we got to the point where were we could almost predict when he would reflux. Compare this to what a physician observes seeing him for a brief time, maybe 15 to 30 minutes a visit. So there was obviously some information we knew that the rest of the team didn't.

On the other hand, there was a lot that the medical team knew that we didn't. With that in mind, what we would do was blend and share the information to try to get the most complete picture of Benjamin's health that we could.

Look for ideas in unusual places. Reflux and GERD are complex problems, and the solutions are not necessarily simple. Between what you know about your baby and what your medical team knows about GER and GERD, a solution may be at hand . . . maybe. Often solutions, especially concerning some of the finer points of GERD, may not be found on a short and simple path. For instance, we received some excellent advice from our lawyer and his wife who had an infant with reflux. Our chiropractor and pharmacist also had wonderful insights, along with our dentist. They helped us see patterns and ask questions that helped us clarify our thoughts. Even our veterinarian was helpful. He reminded us of the importance of the voice of the caregiver who is caring for those who cannot speak.

You need to be careful about the information you receive since sometimes it might not be appropriate or even healthy. So be prudent, and check any ideas with your medical team.

(And be extremely cautious about questionable sources of information on the Internet.)

Communicate clearly. This is absolutely critical to being a great boss, yet few folks communicate well—especially when they are sleep deprived and are reacting to their baby's suffering. In a doctor's office, where time is very limited, and conversations are often brief, each word counts. If you find that your current level of frustration and exhaustion (or any other factor) will prevent you from communicating clearly, try something simple like having a friend make notes of his observations of what is going on and present them to the physician, or bring the friend with you to the appointment. This bit of objectivity might help clarify to the physician what is happening.

And communication is a two-way interaction. Be sure to listen carefully and be very detail oriented. It almost goes without saying that you should take notes at each of your appointments since a great amount of information is often covered in a short amount of time, while you are trying to hold an impatient patient!

Set realistic expectations. One of the early expectations we had was that Benjamin would get healthy quickly. That turned out to be very unreasonable. Even as Ben celebrated his first birthday, reflux was a very big part of his and our lives.

When Ben didn't get well quickly, we had to shift our expectations. Now we expect that he will have a normal life somewhere down the line, and that slowly, but surely, he and we will be able to manage his reflux.

Another expectation you should have about your relationship with your health-care team is that you should be able to get the answers to the questions that you feel that you need answers to. However, like in any employment situation, you need to allow them the time that it may take to get back to you with the needed information. These folks are under a lot of pressure with regards to their time. A good approach is to tell them that you have some questions regarding your child's diagnosis and treatment, and ask them how and when they would prefer that they are asked, and what would be a realistic time for those questions to be answered.

Improve yourself. A good boss improves himself. A common theme in almost any educational environment is to get smart. You work daily to improve yourself. You do homework, you read, solve problems, and do other assorted things to get smarter.

Why is it then when faced with a situation like a medical problem, many parents fold up? Why do they forget all of their educational training? It is important that you educate yourself daily about your baby's health.

Know yourself and your medical team. Be true to yourself and be who you are. For example, if you are an assertive person, and that puts your medical team on edge, or the team doesn't respond well to you, then you need to change your medical team. Or if you are a mild-mannered person, and you feel that you are being pushed, then make a change. Be aware of what is going on and be true to yourself.

Advocate for your people. Dr. Kim Clabaugh, who wrote the foreword for this book, is a veterinarian who has made her living advocating for beings who can't speak, who can't use words to express their pain, their discomfort, their problems.

Your job is no different than hers when you are the parent of an infant with reflux. They can't use words to communicate, so they cry. And you need to take that communication and turn it into words so you can be an advocate for your child. By being a parent, you've got the job of being an advocate, and you have got to do your job.

Be adaptable. Part of being a parent is being adaptable. You invited a new person into your life. That means extra jobs to do and a lot more work. Magnify that five or ten fold when you have an infant with reflux.

We've found over the first year that our life is one of continually being flexible. At a moment's notice our plans get changed, because Ben gets sick or we need to do things to keep him healthy. With two children there was actually a time when we had ten doctors appointments in ten days. When those ten days began we had none. Flexibility is crucial.

Letting go. There will probably come a point in your search for the best health for your baby that you'll need to let go. You will have to trust your medical team or other advisors. If you've done all your homework this will hopefully feel right.

One of the times that really hit us was when they had heard something in Benjamin's lungs and they wanted to check for aspirations, due to the worry about pneumonia. So they said they wanted to take a chest x-ray. This is the first time we had ever been through that process and we said, "Sure, no problem." We both had had x-rays before, and compared to some of Ben's other testing, we thought the X-ray would be simple. Not quite.

With an infant, a chest x-ray is dramatically different. They don't just lie on a table. They are put on a seat in a bike-like contraption, and the poor child, with arms above head, is squeezed between two pieces of round plastic, unable to move. It looks like the worst carnival ride that you can imagine and seeing our screaming infant in there about stopped our hearts (see the picture below).

So here is Ben screaming as loud as he could, frightened to death, and we had to trust. We had to let go.

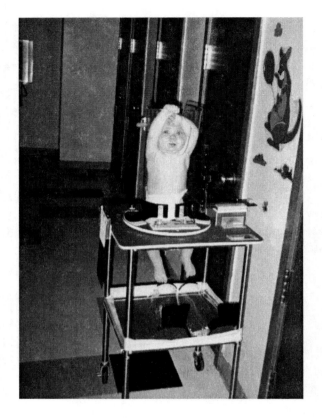

Benjamin preparing for a chest X-ray. He is enclosed in a
plastic tube that forces his arms above his head.

Take care of the details. Being a good boss also means that
you must take care of the details, like such items as payments
and paperwork. Oftentimes you are asking a group of professionals to go beyond their usual call of duty. Be fair with
them. Make sure that you are keeping up with your payments
and any other behind-the-scenes task that makes you a good
boss.

Respect. There needs to be mutual respect between you and the medical team. You have to respect the doctor. He or she must be able to intervene if things are not going well, and that is truly what is meant by being "under a doctor's care."

There may be a time when your doctor recommends something that you are not comfortable with at first. At that point it will come down to trust and respect as to whether or not you take his or her advice.

After many months of inadequate medical care, our *new* pediatric gastroentrologist, at Georgetown University, wanted to admit Ben to the hospital for further testing. While we were terrified of further heartache, from all accounts this doctor was wonderful, and we needed to trust him (with his help, he was able to pinpoint the severity of Ben's reflux and to refer us for surgical and allergy consults).

This respect is a two-way process. Most worthy doctors will realize that for you to have made it this far with this situation, you must be an exceptional parent. That doctor will also know that because you are with that child more than anyone else, you have information that the other team members don't have. They need to respect you and not be threatened by an inquisitive parent who is working hard to help his or her child.

Just keep in mind that respect should not be confused with abdication. Respect means you listen and regard someone as a professional. Respect does not mean that you blindly go along, fearful of questions, afraid to voice your opinion, unwilling to get the answers you need.

Have a good sense of humor. More than likely you'll have some dark nights and days ahead of you. As a boss, finding humor when and where you can might make things a little better.

Evaluate. Evaluating how things are progressing with your baby's treatment is a simple step that quite often is not done, yet it is critical in terms of seeing if your medical team is on track and your baby is getting better.

Here is what we did whenever we began a new course of treatment for Ben. We would do an assessment at the pre-treatment and then again post-treatment (or after a period of time). We evaluated if things had improved.

For example, one benchmark we would use is how Ben slept at night. There was a period of time when Benjamin would wake up every 20 minutes, and was only sleeping about 5 to 6 hours per day—total. So when we began a new treatment we made sure that we had solid records of his sleep pre-treatment. And then we tracked again after two weeks or so. In this case, by a change of medications, we saw a great improvement in his sleep. So our evaluation showed that we were on the right track.

When you evaluate, use objective criteria (facts), and take the subjectivity (fuzzy things) out of it. Items like how many times the baby vomits per day, how many ounces he eats, or how many times he wakes up during his sleep are objective criteria that can help you evaluate. For example "woke seven times" is more factual than "slept poorly," and "cried one hour" is more specific than "was miserable."

HOW TO GET THE MOST FROM THIS STEP

Are They <u>Really</u> Working for You?

Problem: You need to determine if your health-care team is on track with your needs.

Determining if they are *really* working for you can be problematic for several reasons. First, if you have an ill child, this is probably a fairly emotional time for you—and that can make clear judgment and communication difficult. Second, some in the medical profession have a tough time relating to parents (especially upset parents) about what may seem like simple issues such as sleeping and eating. Third, some in the medical profession (especially at teaching hospitals) are biased by their own research—causing them to make biased judgments. For instance, if a physician is researching behavioral issues then that doctor will probably be more prone to suspect behavioral causes over mechanical causes.

In a recent issue of the PAGER newsletter Dr. Sears, a noted pediatrician, reflected about this specific topic:

> I would see babies six and nine months old who had been to four or five different physicians. "Colic," "Worried Mother," "over-reactive," all kinds of misdiagnoses. The worst I heard was letting the baby cry it out. I had mothers come in and we would do an esophagoscopy and find ulcers practically burned through the baby's esophagus wall. The poor moms had been told to let the baby cry it out because they were "spoiling" the baby.[xiv]

All right, back to the problem at hand. How do you find out if they really are working for you, since that actually is not the type of question that you point-blank ask someone?

Here are a few suggestions to help you tease out the answer.

Suggestion 1: Research. Okay—three important parts here. First, is your health-care team up on the current research? Do they know about current trends, studies, and types of treatments? How can you find out if they are? Well, you can ask them. That's one way. Another is to compare their recommendations, treatments, and prescriptions to those from other doctors (support groups can help with this).

Second, do they support you as a member of the team? As we note in the upcoming chapter, *Step 5: Research It to the Bone,* many patients or parents are doing a significant amount of their own research about their or their child's illnesses. To them this is an important part of their healing process. Other patients don't care to do their own research, which is fine. So, does your health-care team support the role that you would like to play in getting your child better?

Third, is your health-care team doing their own research on a topic (or anything) that might be a conflict of interest? For instance, a physician who is treating patients with GERD, but who is also receiving grant money to investigate a type of child abuse such as Munchausen Syndrome by Proxy (MSBP) stands a good chance of having conflicting interests that could be devastating.

For instance, *Family Practice News* reported that at a recent conference, Dr. Jay A. Perman, chairman of the department of pediatrics at the University of Maryland in Baltimore, urges colleagues to begin considering a diagnosis of Munchausen Syndrome by Proxy when they find themselves thinking, "I have never seen anything like this before."[xv]

Suggestion 2: Are you better off? There is one telltale item that can really give you an insight into whether your team is working for you and really how well they are doing. Answer this question, and you'll have your insight:

> Is the quality of my life, and my child's life, better now than it was before we began work-ing with our current health-care team?

When Benjamin turned seven months old we asked that exact same question. The answer came from both of us at exactly the same time . . . a no-hesitation no-doubt-about-it "NO!" Benjamin's quality of life was much worse and so was ours, and it seemed to be getting worse almost weekly. It was at that point that we made a health-care team change. Now we ask that question almost weekly, and we are blessed because so far the answer has been a rousing "YES!"

Suggestion 3: Gut check. If neither of the previous sugges-tions offer any insight, try this . . . do a *gut check*. In sports we use that term to signify when an athlete has reached a point in training or competition when he or she must assess if things are right on track. Well, you do the same, and listen to the an-swer.

So ask yourself, "Are things on track?" "Do I feel that my health-care team is working for me and my family?" And as we said, listen to the answers.

[xii] Reflux Digest. (Summer, 2002. V 6, N 1). <u>Rebecca's story.</u> p.7.

[xiii] Reflux Digest (Spring/Summer, 2001. V 5, N 1). <u>Lucas' Story.</u> p.16.

[xivxiv] Reflux Digest. (Summer, 2002. V 6, N 1). <u>Interview with Bill Sears, MD.</u> p. 4.

[xv] Bates, B. (April, 2000). Flags for munchausen syndrome by proxy. <u>Family Practice News</u>.

Step 5

Research It to the Bone

A while ago we promised to discuss several crucial things that we have unearthed along the way—items that could be incredibly important to you and the care that your child gets. Well, here is one, and it's a big one:

You will need to research, and research like crazy, about what is going on with your child.

Simply enough, research is the act of seeking truth, information, or knowledge about something. There is a wealth of reasons why you should research, and we're going to go into those in a moment. However, before that, we want to discuss one reason that you might *not* want to do any research.

Why You Might Not Want to Research

It appears that there are some (how many we do not know) in the medical community who prefer that their patients do no research. These health-care professionals would rather that their patients, or in this case parents/guardians of their patients, not read or investigate their child's illness and treatment.

We bumped into several of those folks, and the only sound reason that we can infer for this line of thinking is one of control. Some people just want to be in total control . . . information is power . . . power is control. So keep in mind that doing research when you have a doctor like this usually leads to friction.

Eight Reasons Why You Should Research

On the other hand, there are doctors who want you to research, to know all that you can about the illness and treatments. One such doctor is David Cosenza, who had this to say about patients doing research:

> I try to help my patients become educated, and I encourage them to learn more on their own.
> Many of us do more research before we buy a new car than we do about our own personal health.[xv]

And since we are obviously in agreement with Dr. Cosenza, here are eight sensible reasons why you should research acid reflux and GERD, and research them to the bone.

Reason #1: Reflux and GERD are complicated conditions. For example, the support and advocacy group PAGER and some medical experts suspect that reflux might actually be several separate diseases and these diseases are on the frontier of medicine. That means that new information is being published every day. In the course of your research you might be the one to see something that sounds very close to your situation and that you may want to discuss with your doctor.

Reason #2: The more you know, the better decisions you can make. Keeping yourself educated on the latest information may make a big difference in your treatment options. For example, even though a doctor that we respected very much recommended that we consider surgery for Ben, our research led us to a very progressive group at the University of Missouri that was trying different approaches to the disease. Because of our research we were able to consult with this group as an alternative to surgery.

Reason #3: You can double-check the information that you are receiving from your health-care professionals. This can be especially helpful when a variety of medications are simultaneously prescribed.

Reason #4: Education can help you speak the same language as your teammates. Understanding the common terminology of GER and GERD can save everyone time.

Reason #5: Research gives you needed confidence in what may be going on. The health-care team that we worked with at the University of Missouri recommended that we visit the web site of the pH probe manufacturer. Benjamin was going to have the probe inserted surgically and the Missouri team understood that the more we knew about what they would be doing to Benjamin, the better we would feel about it.

Reason #6: Research might help reduce the emotional edge. A physician only has a limited amount of time to spend with you and explain what may be occurring. By doing your own research you can take as much time as you need to understand what the doctor has told you. In our case this helped reduce our stress.

Reason #7: If you are recommended to a new doctor research can help you to check the qualifications of the referred physician.

Reason #8: Research can facilitate your understanding of what you will be discussing at your next appointment, and therefore help you to be better prepared to ask specific questions and make better use out of the limited time that you have with your doctor.

This quote by Beth Anderson, the head of PAGER, might help put the importance of research into perspective for you:

> Unfortunately, changes in the actual treatment of reflux are always a little slower in coming to the public. This is why I always recommend that parents do all they can to educate themselves and keep up with the research that is coming out. Many doctors don't stay current or tend to be wary of the newest treatments but for patients who are not doing well with *older treatments*, it is up to the parents to be constantly on the look-out for promising new ideas.[xvi]

My, How Things Have Changed

Back in the 1880s physicians did not exist as we know them today. People cared for most of their own health problems, and they had complete access to any and all medical tools and treatments available at that time.[xvii] That changed in the 1900s, when a physician-centered health-care system developed. And with that came a dramatic shift with medical tools and treatments becoming the sole property of physicians.

This physician-centered ownership kept evolving unhindered until around the late 1960s, when people slowly started to want more control of their health care. This was in part driven by the spirit of those revolutionary years, and also by a crisis in health care due to skyrocketing costs.

This change in ownership was reflected by the seminal book *Our Bodies, Ourselves*, which Dr. Tom Ferguson noted was "the prototype for a new generation of medical guides . . . which would enable them [readers] to play a more responsible role in managing their own health care."

Since then the change has been continuing to evolve. Ferguson, who is known for his work on the development of online health resources and "e-patients" (http://www.doctom.com), wrote that by the 1990s, "The age of unquestioned 'doctor's orders' has been replaced by an era of 'shared medical decision-making.'"[xviii]

Today, Ferguson's research has found that more than six million people consult online health resources every day, which he noted to be more than twice as many as the number who consult physicians.[xix]

That's a lot of people who are researching. Shouldn't you be one?

How to Get It Done

There is a wealth of resources out there on the topic of research. The one book we have found to be the most helpful about researching has been *A Guide to Research for Educators and Trainers of Adults*, by Merriam and Simpson (1995). We are not advocating that you find a copy and jump into it, un-less of course you have a lot of free time. But since you probably don't, let us distill the book into one simple concept that the authors impart about research:

> They defined research as "a systematic process by which we know more about something than we did before engaging in the process."

Simple enough. However, the part that seems to cause people the most problem is this "systematic process." So let us help.

When we advocate research, we are in essence suggesting that you read, in an organized fashion, articles and books that are relevant to what is happening. There are numerous research-ers, many graduate students and medical researchers, who are conducting investigations almost daily into GERD and reflux. What you need to do is locate their reports and see what con-clusions they might have drawn. We also advocate that you search the Web, using a search engine, and use e-mail to seek information and solicit support from peers, friends, family, and support groups.

To help you get going with your research, see the section at the end of this chapter. However, before you do that, please read the following.

Be Careful—Very, Very Careful

At best, research might:

➢ offer you insight into the disease your child has,

➢ expose you to possible treatment steps to consider,

➤ reveal new thoughts on the illness, and/or

➤ provide suggestions for home care efforts.

However, if you're not careful your research can make things . . . well . . . worse.

How can it make things worse? Well, if the information is bad it can:

➤ lead to unwise decisions,

➤ be emotionally unsettling,

➤ waste valuable time, and/or

➤ be totally wrong.

And if your physician is not supportive of your researching the problem, difficulties and friction can arise in your relationship. Any of those things may make your situation more complicated. To help avoid them, we submit these following suggestions for you to contemplate:

First, consider your source. Locating information today is significantly easier than it has ever been, in large part due to the Web. It almost seems as if the information is ready to jump right out at you. Take the utmost care when getting any information from the Web, and use only reputable sources. Be mindful that the information is only as reliable as the source.

Second, don't generalize. If you are reading studies or reviews of experiments realize that almost all findings are not applicable outside of the sample group that was used for the research.

Third, use common sense when you get information. We suggest that you use appropriate information you find as material for discussion with your medical team. We strongly, strongly, strongly caution you to not make any changes to your child's treatment or care until you have conferred with your team.

Fourth, if you are researching, you are going to be changing your relationship with your physician from the traditional provider-centered system to a new patient-centered system (as Dr. Ferguson calls it). Make sure your health-care provider is on board with this.

And more than anything else, keep this one thought in mind:

If something sounds too good to be true, it probably is.

So often, people buy things or try things because they believe that there is a miracle cure handy. Seldom, seldom, seldom does that ever work out well.

And one final cautionary thought—be skeptical. Authors Merriam and Simpson[xx] noted that rarely does anyone track down the original raw data of studies to check the accuracy of the findings—meaning that the findings presented might not be correct.

HOW TO GET THE MOST FROM THIS STEP

How to Research

Problem: You're here because you need information about what is going on.

Needed: Telephone, access to the Web, note-taking material, library access.

There once was a fisherman who made his living by going out each morning, casting his net into the ocean, and bringing his catch back to sell at the dock. He made a good living because he knew four things. First, he knew *why* he was fishing. Second, he knew *what* type of fish that people were going to buy each day. Third, he knew *where* he could find those fish on a specific day. And fourth, he knew *how* to fish.

Before you begin any quest for information, think of yourself as that fisherman. Your quest will be much more productive if you know: (1) why you are looking for information, (2) what knowledge you are looking for, (3) where the best place is to find the information, and (4) how to find it.

Let's take a closer look at the why, what, where, and how of researching reflux and GERD.

Step 1: Why and what? The why is fairly simple: you are trying to improve the quality of life for you, your child, and your entire family. Exactly what information you are looking for is going to be a little bit harder to determine because that may change on a day-to-day basis, not unlike what fish people

87

are buying. For instance, one day you may want to know something like, "What exactly is a Tucker Sling?" and the next day you might want to know, "When will this all get better?" Pin down your *what* before you begin researching. It will keep you from getting overwhelmed and sidetracked.

Step 2: Where to look. Now we're getting to the tricky part. Where do you turn for answers to your *what*? We have identified seven sources of information that we use. Here they are in alphabetical order:

> ➢ Articles
> ➢ Friends in the medical community
> ➢ Friends/family with reflux
> ➢ Parents of kids with reflux
> ➢ Studies
> ➢ Support groups
> ➢ Websites

Each one of those areas has given us a wealth of information that has helped us improve the quality of our and Ben's life. For example:

From this source:	We learned such things as:
Articles	The lay person's view of GERD and reflux.
Friends in the medical community	To push hard to find solutions.
Friends/family with reflux	That the pain can be horrific, that reflux keeps many people awake much of the night, that a drink of water can help immensely during an episode.
Parents of children with reflux	That certain foods may make reflux worse, that reflux can cause many other problems (i.e., asthma).
Academic studies	The medical and experts' view of GER and GERD.
Support groups	So many other parents were sharing our experiences.
Web sites	Potential reaction to some medications, research that our medical team was involved in.

Step 3: Now for the <u>how</u>. We tend to be very simplistic in our research, in that we basically have broken the *how* down into two methods: We ask questions and we read a lot.

<u>Ask Questions</u>. A very important part of research that many folks overlook is that of asking questions. We have asked, and probably will keep on asking until Benjamin is cured, an enormous amount of questions. And interestingly enough, the answers to those questions often lead to other questions whose answers can be critical.

For instance, we were discussing Ben's condition with a friend who happened to be a pathologist. Her child had reflux. Very early into Benjamin's illness we told her that he had been diagnosed with *colic*, and asked her what would she do, if this was her child. Her words still ring in our ears today. She said, "Well, I wouldn't stop there!" That advice prompted us to find out more, and we found out that Benjamin had *GERD*, which we had never heard of before. And that advice stayed with us through the entire process. One simple question delivered an answer that had a major impact.

<u>Read</u>. A few years back we were browsing through a used book store. We came upon a book entitled *How to Read a Book*. After initially scoffing at the title, we opened it up, and we've got to say, it's a good book—really good—and they have sold a multitude of copies of it since its original printing in 1940.

So what does that have to do with reflux research? Well the authors, Adler and Van Doren, identified three types of reading: reading for entertainment, reading for information, and reading for understanding. The authors noted that doing research using the last two types of reading is the most effective.

Reading for information and/or understanding is an active process. Reading for entertainment is passive, and many folks get into difficulty when researching when they try to research like they read for entertainment. Basically, how you skim the *TV Guide* doesn't work well for reading scientific articles.

Look at it this way, when you are researching you are trying to gain information from people who know more than you. If you asked a person a question, he or she would usually give you an answer—pretty easy. However, when you read with a question in mind you must answer it yourself, and that takes work. Today, most scientific writings are written for experts by experts. That means that you really have two choices when researching.

The first choice is *scientific popularizations*, such as magazine and newspaper articles. The information in them is usually presented in an easy reading manner, which might make digesting the material easier. While these are great beginner researching resources, you will be at the mercy of reporters who filter the information for you.

The second choice is *scientific articles*. These are often dry and lengthy. However, reviewing the articles and focusing on the abstract and discussion sections may offer you some valuable insight. Also, a review of the reference section might be enlightening.

One very important part of reading for research is note taking. We're not going to get into that here, but let us say that if you read something applicable or of interest then you should write it down—because it can easily disappear. Another important part is to achieve an understanding of what you are reading before you begin to criticize or assess significance.

Finding items to read shouldn't be difficult—the nearest source of medical literature is really no further away than the nearby computer and Internet connection. Here is an example of how to do it:

1) Find a computer with Internet access and go to http://www.google.com.
2) Where it asks you to "search," put in the signs that you are observing in your child, for example, you might put in "crying, choking, and spitting up."
3) Hit return. You will probably see pages and pages of information. Just scan this information, knowing that as you gain more information about your child's condition, some of these articles may become more meaningful.
4) Read away. But remember, be cautious of the source you are using.
5) To further fine-tune your research, click on the "Advance Search" button, and follow the guidelines. Try a variety of key words such as *colic*, *vomiting*, and *gagging*, and see what you get.
6) Be aware that rarely will you find the full text of a medical article on-line; instead comprehensive summaries are often offered. If you find a "must-have" article, then take the specific reference information to your nearest library and request a copy of the article.

[xv] Bridges. (Spring 2003, V 4, N 4). <u>A new face in Centreville.</u> p. 6.

[xvi] Anderson, B., & Anderson, L. (1992). Practical hints on caring for babies with reflux. Unpublished manuscript.

[xvii] Ferguson, T (in press). What e-patients can teach us about health care reform. E-Patients, Online Health, and the Search for Sustainable Healthcare

[xviii]. Ibid

[xix] Ibid

[xx] Merriam, S., & Simpson, E. (1995). A guide to research for educators and trainers of adults. Malabar, FL: Krieger Publishing Company.

Step 6

With a Little Help from Your Friends

Little doubt about it, our first year with Benjamin was one of the hardest physical and mental things we had ever done. We had both participated in college sports and this was much tougher. There is no way that we could have done it without support—a lot of support—from our family, friends, and acquaintances.

When we first became aware of Benjamin's illness we were hesitant to ask for help outside of the medical profession. This was for a couple of reasons. One, for example, was our sense of pride—we felt like we should be able to handle this, especially when we were often told that it was just a "little bit" of reflux. Another was that we didn't have a clue how bad his illness was and the effect it would have on us. And yet another was that we didn't want to burden people with our problems. However, six months into the process, our physical and mental condition dictated to us to ask for help.

You see, life before a new baby is a lot like driving a brand new car down the road on a nice, straight highway. You can pretty much go where you want, when you want to. However, when you add a new healthy baby to your family you can still keep on driving, although for a while it's going to be difficult to keep going without some stops here and there. However, when you have a baby with acid reflux it is like someone is constantly putting the parking brake on. You go nowhere, and nowhere fast. And that was actually our family's code name for a really bad day with Ben; we would say that we had been "Braked!"

Our yard was a mess, our garden looked like a bomb had gone off in it, and it seemed like an F3 tornado had touched down inside our house. Our cars were hanging on by a thread and we missed bill deadlines left and right. We looked and felt terrible and were grossly sleep deprived. Our two small businesses were greatly affected. Our number one son was definitely playing second fiddle as we spent most of our time caring for Ben. And our jobs . . . well, let's just say that we were very lucky to have understanding bosses and seniority at both of our jobs. And lucky to keep our jobs.

Yup, our life had gone to hell in a hand basket and it became apparent that it was time to call in the cavalry. The first to respond were our families, second our friends, and third our coworkers. In short time we had frequent dinners being made for us, folks helping with our eldest son, people spending the night once a week so we could sleep, and people helping out in more ways than we could ever imagine. The difference it made was very significant.

Well, that was us. How about you? Should you ask people for help, more help than you have now? That is what the task at the end of this chapter is all about.

HOW TO GET THE MOST FROM THIS STEP

Do You Need Support?

Problem: Your life is being turned upside down. Do you need to call in the cavalry?

This exercise can serve two purposes. Not only can you see the areas in your life that may need more attention, but it can also lead you in a conversation with family members about what is, or isn't, a priority in your life right now while you have a high-needs baby.

Sometimes it helps just to have such a conversation with your partner about what is important now and what is not. Such discussions can give each other permission to let go of some of the stress, or it can let your partner and/or family know the areas that really mean a lot to you, and those areas can become more of a focus.

Step 1: Do you need the cavalry? If you have a child with acid reflux you can and should get assistance from your health-care team to diagnose and treat the illness. Just how complicated the reflux is will determine if you need support in other areas of your life. For example, Benjamin's case was (and still is) complex and as noted in this chapter we needed a lot of help.

To determine if you might need more support than you already have we have included a simple chart. You will find multiple areas that tend to get neglected when intensive childcare is required. To use the chart, circle the appropriate number that represents the current condition of an area as compared to how it was before your baby with reflux. (Feel free to put other areas in; the ones listed were affected the greatest in our life). Here is an example:

> What is the condition of your sense of humor now, compared to before your baby with acid reflux?

Much Worse	Somewhat Worse	Same	Somewhat Better	Much Better
1	2	3	4	5

1) How does the interior of your house look now, compared to before your baby with acid reflux?

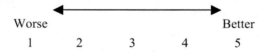

	Worse				Better	
	1	2	3	4	5	

2) How are your cars running now, compared to before your baby with acid reflux?

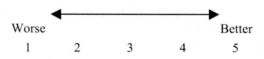

	Worse				Better	
	1	2	3	4	5	

3) Compared to before your baby with reflux, how healthy are you eating?

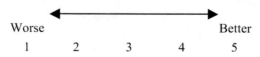

	Worse				Better	
	1	2	3	4	5	

4) How is your sleep now compared to before your baby with acid reflux?

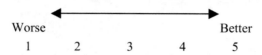

Worse   Better

1   2   3   4   5

5) Your yard looks _____ now, compared to before your baby with reflux.

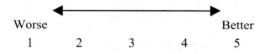

Worse   Better

1   2   3   4   5

6) How are you doing paying your bills?

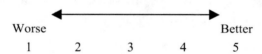

Worse   Better

1   2   3   4   5

7) Your attention to your other child(ren) is _____.

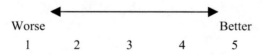

Worse   Better

1   2   3   4   5

8) The quality of time you are spending with your partner is

_____.

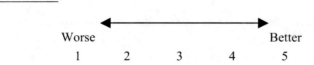

Worse   Better

1   2   3   4   5

9) Compared to before your baby with reflux, how is your stress level?

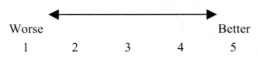

Worse   Better

1   2   3   4   5

10) Your job performance is _____ compared to before your baby with reflux.

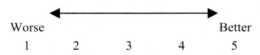

Worse   Better

1   2   3   4   5

Step 2: Determine your score. Add up the numbers that you have circled. Your total is: _____ .

Step 3: In general, how are you doing? Now take your total and compare it to the following:

If your point total is:	*You should:*
10 to 20	Get support, and fast.
21 to 30	Work on getting support as soon as you can.
31 to 50	Pat yourself on the back, because you are doing great.

Step 4: Where do you need specific help? Do you have any 1's? If so, then that particular area is one that you should probably get help in, or make a decision that it is no longer (or temporarily not) a priority. We knew, for instance, that our yard was not getting nearly as much TLC as it was used to,

and it looked pretty bad. Realizing this was a problem area for us, we hired the son of a friend to come over a few times to help. Even a few hours made a great difference in how we felt about things.

Step 5: Whom can you call? Before you sound the alarm and call in the support troops, let us impart this word of warning based on our experiences. We found that the people we knew who had a history with us and who cared about us were the ones who responded quickly and caringly. Be cautious about reaching out to people with whom you don't have a relationship. These people, especially if they have never had a sick child, may misinterpret you or your request for help.

All right, with that out in the open, here are some people and places that you may consider reaching out to:

> *Your Partner:* As simple as this might sound, the first place you should look for support is in your partner. In our case we both worked on Ben's care equally. However, in some relationships this doesn't happen for a variety of reasons (e.g., job constraints).

> *Your Workplace:* Make full use of your sick leave and to help that happen you may want to make sure that your supervisor understands exactly what you are going through (this may require medical documentation). Also, you may find your coworkers more sympathetic than you can imagine, since many adults suffer from acid reflux.

Family: You may or may not have family members in a position to help. If you do, welcome their assistance.

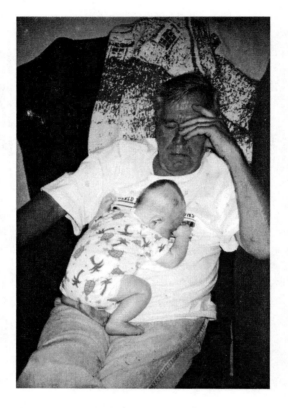

A part of our cavalry, Grandfather rests after a long day.

Support Groups: There are support groups for just about any situation you can imagine. For children with GER and GERD there are probably several, but the one we found to be of won-

derful help is a group in Maryland called
PAGER (http://www.reflux.org).

Friends: If you decide to approach your friends
you will probably be as surprised at their reac-
tions as we were. We had some friends who
were so supportive that it just blew us away;
and we even found some friends whose children had had similar problems when they were
babies (those were the folks who were always
holding Benjamin while we ate.) At the other
end of the spectrum, we found some friends
who we assumed were going to be helpful and
supportive but who weren't and just disappeared. For them, it was just beyond their ca-
pacity to help.

Babysitters: It used to be that you hired a babysitter and then vacated the premises—went out
to a dinner or a movie. We found that we had to
hire a babysitter just so we could pick up
around the house or spend time with our other
child (we were terrified to ever leave the house
for more than one hour).

Church: Most churches have some type of a
caring committee for families in need. If you
belong to a church, be sure to let the appropriate people at your church know what is happening.

Making Life Better —

Step 7

Recharge Your Batteries

Back in the early 1970s the United States went through a pretty tough time called the *Energy Crisis*. As a country we were consuming more energy than we produced so we had to import it. The folks we were importing it from decided they weren't going to give us any more and whammo, we had a crisis. Well, if you are not careful as a caregiver of a child with acid reflux you may well suffer your own energy crisis.

Caring for a child with a disability or chronic illness can have a profound effect on the caregiver. When parents treat children with special health-care needs such as reflux, they begin a process that can be accompanied by periods of stress, uncertainty, and feelings of overwhelming loneliness and isolation. Following is a true story from parents of a chronically ill child taken from the National Information Center for Children and Youth with Disabilities (NICHCY) Web site (http://www.nichcy.org) to help describe what we mean.

> Of the first six months of my child's life, three and a half months were spent in the hospital. We lived in a world of intensive care, with car-

diac monitors, oxygen tents, tubes in every ori-
fice and IV's in every extremity of my daughter's body.

The weeks my daughter was home were completely taken up with her care: two hours to get
a meal in her, so for six hours a day I was
feeding her; up many nights holding her so she
could sleep on my shoulder so that she could
breathe if she had a respiratory infection. Respiratory infections were frequent because of her
disabilities, and many nights my husband and I
would have to get our older child up, take him
to our neighbor's house and take my daughter
to the hospital where she could have oxygen if
her breathing got too labored. After getting her
admitted, we would go back home, and get up
again the next morning to get our son off to
school and to return to the hospital. This after
being awakened in the middle of the night with
a phone call from the hospital saying that they
were transferring her to intensive care so she
could be watched more closely.

During that time, either my husband or I always
had to be with our daughter while the other ran
to the grocery, the bank, the pediatrician for our
son's health-care needs, or just to sleep for a
few hours. Our friends disappeared from our
lives.

As this parent so aptly describes, caring for a chronically ill
child, such as one with acid reflux can quickly drain your en-

ergy. Specifically, your emotional, physical, and spiritual energy. And when that happens, problems can occur unless you have a plan to replace that energy.

Recharging Your Batteries

Many of us like to think that we can run on and on like the Energizer Bunny™. However, as we just discussed, that's not so, and your batteries will run down. (Notice the choice of word: *will* instead of *might*.)

To keep it simple, we like to describe recharging your batteries as finding your emotional, physical, or spiritual center, nourishing your soul, or practicing self-care to maintain your emotional health.

We know from experience that maintaining your emotional health is typically low on the list of daily priorities. So, the challenge in recharging your batteries is to search for sources of renewal in your daily routines (unless you know something we don't, that exotic Caribbean vacation probably isn't happening anytime soon, and we haven't been to both a dinner and a movie since the turn of the century).

In our case, many well-meaning friends, relatives, and caregivers tried to suggest breaks for us that just weren't realistic. Unless you had spent time with Ben, you just didn't have a clue how hard it was to leave him alone. When Tracy visited her mom in Florida, her mother told her to "Go take a break and have some fun." When Tracy returned after only a few hours, Tracy's mom was sitting on her bed, with a screaming baby and said, "It scares me how hard Ben is crying. I don't think I will be able to do that again!" (She has since helped in so many other ways, as grandmothers always do.)

So, to keep it realistic, recharging may be as simple as...

> ➤ Positive self-talk (Since last June, Mike, a professional coach, has walked around the house mumbling, "We can do this, we can do this...")

> ➤ Reading a chapter from a favorite book (notice we had the experience not to suggest the whole book?)

> ➤ Taking a bath and lighting a candle

> ➤ Taking a few minutes for prayer or meditation

> ➤ Having a focused conversation (or e-mail) with a friend

> ➤ Attending one support group meeting (moms' or dads' group or reflux- or feeding-support group, for example)

> ➤ Doing any amount of exercise that you can sneak in

> ➤ Learning something new (Tracy has learned to roller blade 15 minutes at a time since the birth of Benjamin)

Those are some of the recharging activities that we do. Yours may be totally different, and the section at the end of this chapter might help you to discover some of them.

HOW TO GET THE MOST FROM THIS STEP

Recharging Your Batteries

Problem: Your energy supply is dwindling. How might you begin to recharge?

Answer the following questions for valuable insights into ways that you might recharge your batteries.

1) How do you care for yourself each day?

2) What activities give you renewed energy?

3) What activities calm you?

4) If you had just 15 minutes each day, what could you add to your routine to renew your spirit?

5) Pre-kids, what did you do to relax? Can you do something similar?

6) Make a list of quickie relaxers and put them in a conspicuous place for all to see.

Step 8

Stay Healthy

Like many Americans we have both been blessed with relatively good health. Besides the occasional bout with the flu, colds, and the assorted sports-related injuries, our lives have been pretty healthy. That is, until this past year.

Within a period of six months Mike contracted bronchitis (never had it before), our oldest son came down with croup for the first time and had to be rushed to the emergency room, and Tracy had a spell of blurred vision that lasted for quite a while.

We had both become so focused on caring for Benjamin that our own health began to pay the price. This became very evident after one hospital stay in the spring of 2003. After two days of testing and wonderful care at Georgetown University Hospital, the three of us (Tracy, Benjamin, and Mike) came home. By the time we got back, both adults became very sick—ill with strep throat. Now strep throat in itself is not exactly a pleasant experience, but what made it worse was that neither of us, even with treatment of antibiotics, could shake it. It took several return visits to the doctors' offices and long courses of medication to finally recover.

We believe that from lack of sleep our immune systems had become so run down that we became more susceptible to illness. Interestingly enough, there is a significant amount of research that supports just that premise. In fact, there is research that indicates that the stress of care giving may make you considerably more vulnerable to tension, fatigue, irritability, sleep disorders, lethargy, becoming close-minded and inflexible, and questioning your ability to parent. Additionally, the stress may lead to a variety of serious health-related issues such as depression and heart attacks.

What Is Being "Healthy"?

Being "healthy" does not necessarily mean absence of illness. Dr. Weil, well-known advocate of alternative medicine, had this thought to offer on being healthy:

> I believe that the essence of health is balance and a kind of inner resilience that allows you to move through the world and not get hurt by all the things out there that have the potential to injure you. Part of being normally healthy is the cycles our bodies go through, which includes periods of temporary illness or injury, followed by stretches of physical wellness. So you can get the flu and still, on an underlying level, be healthy.[xxi]

So what does all this mean? Well, as we found out, not only will you be caring for an ill child, but your health also may be at risk—that is, unless you take steps to care for yourself—both mentally and physically. Today, most people are inundated with messages about their health from TV, radio, and newsprint.

We are not medical experts, but since you are reading this we realize that you might appreciate our perspective on staying healthy in exceptional times like you might be undergoing.

HOW TO GET THE MOST FROM THIS STEP

Stay Healthy

Problem: How do you, the caregiver, keep as healthy as possible?

Maintaining good health is not a given. A car requires routine maintenance to keep running well, and so does your body. It takes work to stay well. Unfortunately, when there are exceptional demands in our lives we tend to not make routine maintenance a priority.

Caring for a child suffering from acid reflux can be an exceptionally demanding time, and exceptional things can happen. There were nights where we never slept, with Benjamin waking after twenty minutes of sleep and then screaming for hours. There were days when we were so tired, so run down, so off-centered that our health was really in jeopardy. These were very extraordinary times.

Depending on the severity of your child's reflux your health may very well be at risk due to lack of sleep, exposures at doctors' offices, altered eating patterns, chronic stress, and the constant load of carrying a baby, among other reasons. So what's a reasonable parent to do?

Here are a few of our suggestions to be mindful of:

Step 1: This book. Well, first, we suggest that the chapters and steps outlined in this book are a solid place to start. By grasping what might be ahead of you and trying to improve the quality of life as best you can, you hopefully can reduce stress and be better able to care for your child.

Step 2: Your doctor. Often if your child has severe reflux or GERD you will be seeing a specialist such as a gastroentrologist. Keep in contact with your own personal doctor. Make an appointment and inform him or her exactly what is happening in your life. Explain that you have concerns about your own health in this situation.

The physician may be able to make suggestions for your health and he or she may have resources for your family. In Mike's case, his general practitioner had gone through a similar experience with his own child so he was very sensitive to what Mike was experiencing. In fact, often when Mike went to the doctor a significant amount of time was spent talking about Benjamin and what to do to help.

Step 3: Take care of yourself. Weave as much self-care into your daily life as possible. (Notice we did not write "daily routine," since reflux often has a way of dismantling any semblance of a routine.) You might darn well need help to do this. A mentor, friend, guru, instructor, on-line resource, what have you may be able to help. We found some great resources close by, including a yoga instructor and a friend who is a massage therapist.

[xxi] Meaning of health. (2003) http://www.drweil.com/app/-cda/drwCDAQAPrint.html-questionId=3370

Step 9

Be Prepared to Spend Money

This may blow over very quickly—two months from now, this could all be a distant memory. In fact, you may not even have time to get to the bank, and it's over. A majority of kids outgrow reflux before their first birthday.

However, as we write this book, Ben is a year and a half and still has severe reflux, and the financial burdens continue to be great. We are writing this to tell you that there may be a chance that you are going to have to spend a lot of money (even if you have good health insurance) to care for your child with reflux. The full range of costs associated with pediatric GERD has not been studied, nor have the costs associated with lack of treatment.[xxii]

They say that there are two times in your life that you will need more money—when your children are babies, and when they go to college. That piece of advice is oh . . . so . . . pertinent if your child has reflux.

Here are just a few of the increased expenses you might run into:

➢ Medication(s): There are a variety of medications that reflux children are often treated with. (One of our friend's daughters was taking up to 12 medications at the age of 6.)

➢ Formula(s): Oftentimes formulas are changed in an attempt to find one that helps reduce the reflux symptoms. Some formulas can be very expensive and are seldom covered by health insurance.

➢ Doctor and hospital visits: GER is recognized as a chronic condition, which means that you may be seeing a lot of doctors, and that can be expensive—even a simple co-pay can begin to add up. If the reflux is very severe, surgery, and all of the associated expenses, may be necessary.

➢ Babysitters: If you have other young children, it is inevitable that you will need to enlist the help of others to care for them.

➢ Dry cleaning and laundry: If you've got a refluxer who vomits you'll probably be doing a lot of laundry—a whole lot.

➢ Special care items: Babies with reflux often need to sleep on an incline, and to be carried in an upright position. Chances are that you'll need unique items such as a crib that can incline, special carriers, or even a sling-type device to keep the infant positioned appropriately when sleeping.

➤ Legal bills: There is a chance, a slim one, albeit still a
chance, that you might need to engage the services of a
lawyer.

To help you get a picture of the possible cost associated with a
baby with reflux, we thought it might be helpful to highlight
some of our expenses associated with Ben's illness.

In the last 14 months, Ben has had over 50 doctor visits ($10
co-pay each), five different hospital admissions in four different hospitals (the last of which was at the University of Missouri, which meant that we had to fly our other child to his
grandmother's in Florida [$500]), he has taken seven medica-
tions for his reflux (approx. $10 each week), is now on a spe-
cial formula ($60 a week), and due to the misfortune of
spending too much time early on with doctors that didn't
know much about reflux, we have incurred some legal bills.

Of course this accounting doesn't include missed work, or the
cost of the extra help that we have needed to have around the
house, or the special groceries that we are currently buying at
the health food store because his stomach is still so sensitive.

Our purpose in sharing this is not to scare you, but we sure do
wish that we would have known ahead of time what the fiscal
implications of this "Oh-don't-worry-he'll-outgrow-it-in-a-
few-months-just-a-little-bit-of-reflux-looks-fine-to-me-seems-
to-be-thriving" disease were.

HOW TO GET THE MOST FROM THIS STEP

Assessing Your Financial Situation

Problem: Is there a financial disaster looming on your horizon?

As much as some people would like you to believe differently, no one can predict the future, especially when it comes to your finances. However, with a little groundwork, you can get a pretty accurate idea of your current situation and an indication of what the future may bring.

We don't know a great amount about accounting and finances, but there is one thing that we know with absolute certainty. That is, when you have a chronically ill child, your financial situation will change.

Step 1: Seek help. With that thought hanging out there—that your situation will change—one of the best things that you can do for yourself is to seek out the guidance of a financial advisor.

Okay, so you might have a fancy program on your computer that tracks all your money, or a hefty rainy-day fund. So did we, and we got financially rocked. Between the medications, doctor appointments, travel, formulas, etc. the rainy-day fund quickly evaporated and we found ourselves really struggling with the money. One of our saving graces was our accountant. He looked at our finances from a non-emotional perspective and made recommendations that made all the difference in the world.

Step 2: Who are you looking for? We suggest that you seek someone who can perform a current accounting of your finances. This might be an accountant or a financial advisor. Or it might be a friend. Regardless of the title of the person, there are two traits you are looking for. One is trust. Can you and do you trust the person? That is paramount. The other is the person's knowledge. Does he or she know what is necessary to help?

Step 3: What are you looking for? Simply, you are looking for two things. One is the bottom line on personal worth. In particular, what is your worth at this point in time, and what resources do you have available (e.g., cash, equity) if you were to need them? The second is your current money flow. Are you spending more money than you have coming in? Those two items can give you an idea of what your flow is.

Why do you want to know this? Of course, you want to avoid financial disaster. However, you also want to keep your money situation from adding to the stress that you and your family are already experiencing.

Step 4: It's a positive. If the determination is that your flow is positive (income is greater than expenses), great. Keep paying the bills and build up a rainy day fund as much as possible. Financially speaking, what we found with Benjamin was that there were some sunny days; however, there were a lot of rainy days, and there were a few hurricane days with more rain than we had ever seen.

Step 5: It's a wash. If your flow turns out to be zero (income equals expenses) trouble might be just ahead. The main reason is that it doesn't give you much wiggle room in case your money requirements change. So we suggest that you scrimp and save as much as possible and build up a cushion. Why? With reflux, especially severe reflux, complications can occur that need treatment that can be expensive. For instance, Benjamin picked up a stomach virus that in combination with his reflux was terrible. That put him in the hospital for six days.

Assume the best, and plan for the worst.

Step 6: It's a negative. If your flow is negative (income is less than expenses), trouble is here. Sooner or later, probably sooner, there will be a reckoning. At this point we cannot recommend strongly enough to get assistance and develop a plan.

Don't turn a blind eye to this. Even if you're an optimist, if your child has reflux, you've got enough stress in your life. You don't need money issues to compound that stress. So to keep the stress from building, we suggest that you take positive steps as soon as you can, and get someone, and it may be the person who helped you determine your flow, to help you with a plan.

We had to do this, and our accountant presented several things that needed to be done. We had to make some very difficult choices, but those choices made an enormous difference in our stress level, helping us avoid financial disaster.

Two of those choices involved our retirement plans. We decided that Tracy would make early withdraws from her account, whereas I would stop making contributions to mine. Both steps increased our available cash and really made a difference.

In addition to having a financial mentor, you can also take simple steps such as cutting coupons, asking doctors for samples, and working with your insurance company to pay for special formulas.

[xxii] Reflux Digest. (June 2003. V7, N2) <u>PAGER testifies before congress.</u> p. 4.

Step 10

It's Not Over Until It's Over

D
r. Jeff Phillips from the University of Missouri says, "Reflux comes in waves." One of the things that has become very clear to us about reflux is that "it's not over until it's over."

We found that just about the time that Ben would adjust to a new medication, it would stop working, or just about the time that a new medication would appear to have the reflux and nighttime choking under control, he would appear to be having seizure-type episodes each time he fell asleep. It then seemed that once his medication would be under control, he would begin cutting teeth, or even worse, contract the rotavirus, or let's not even mention the introduction of solid food and the associated repercussions.

Hopefully, this won't be your situation, but we do want you to be aware ahead of time that some days you may feel like you have conquered all, just to find out that the constant acid baths have caused an enormous amount of erosion on your baby's new teeth, or that the continuous reflux is creating numerous ear infections.

Patience Is Definitely Going to Be Needed

While a lot has been learned about treating reflux, there is no cure, and there really isn't always a complete understanding of what the disease is. Your final treatment may involve some *art* versus *science*—the solution may be 80% science, and the last 20% may be art (this is one of the reasons that you want to work with someone with a lot of reflux knowledge and experience: to improve the art part). Because of the art part, it requires patience—our baby had a reaction to two very common medications and that has required several doctors to experiment with dosages and medications. This has taken months to perfect (unlike, say, a sinus infection for which you can almost always count on a single prescription of medication to do the trick).

You Must Be Vigilant

As the caregiver, you are closest to your child, which means that you must be vigilant, even though this thing may go on for a while longer than you had hoped. And there are three aspects to vigilance.

First, changes to your child's health can be subtle and can happen almost unbeknownst to you. These changes may come in the form of the baby waking up three times a night, then four times, and before you know it you are back to being up 12 times a night because your child has just been through a growth spurt and has outgrown the present dosage of medication.

Second, since you are the one closest to your child, you will be in a position to see things that your health-care provider won't be able to see.

Third, you know the complete history of your child and can be the one to connect the dots that others might not. For instance, Ben was given his normal immunizations at the beginning of a week by his pediatrician. Later in the week his GI specialist thought that he looked very pale and he was given a blood test to check for an infection. The test came back as strongly positive. After some head scratching we thought that there might be a possible connection between the test results and the recent shots, and it turned out that there probably was.

Endurance

No matter what the complexity, pediatric gastroesophageal reflux is an endurance test for the entire family. Because the challenges seem to just keep on coming, it might be a good idea to enlist the help of a therapist. We have found a great guy who has the experience of someone in his family being sick, and knows the day-to-day pressure that situation can create.

We have asked him very specifically to be a part of Ben's treatment team, by helping us not only to keep our anxiety in check, but also to give us the strength and encouragement to go the extra mile to get Ben the best care that we can manage (he was key in supporting our trip to the University of Missouri, which made a huge difference in the quality of Ben's life). This has involved meeting with him every few weeks and going over what has transpired with Ben, including any medical test results. This helps us keep on an emotional even keel, keep things in perspective, and have the emotional strength to be proactive.

Current research suggests that many affected children outgrow most or all of their symptoms of reflux between the ages of 1 and 5 years old [xxiii]. However, you don't know when that might happen for your child. It could be one year, it could be five years, or it could be never. In fact, some persons are affected into adulthood.

The Power of You

Jon Kabat-Zinn, in his book *Full Catastrophe Living*, writes:

> There is an art to facing difficulties in ways that lead to effective solutions. When we are able to mobilize our inner resources to face our problems artfully, we find we are usually able to orient ourselves in such a way that we can use the pressure of the problem itself to propel us through it, just as a sailor can position a sail to make the best use of the pressure of the wind to propel itself.[xxiv]

This may be a long haul for you and your family. You are the one that can make the greatest difference in the quality of life for your child, your family, and you. According to Dr. Sears,

> I mention to parents that it is important for them to feel like valuable members of the medical team, because the treatment of GER is primarily parental intensive care. That is an important

message that parents need to understand. GER is not anything that any medicine is completely going to fix.[xxv]

Chronic pain demands a proactive mind-set. You need to help yourself at a time when all you want is for someone to save you. Believe in yourself, and trust your instincts if you think that something is wrong with your child, don't give up, and believe in the power of you.

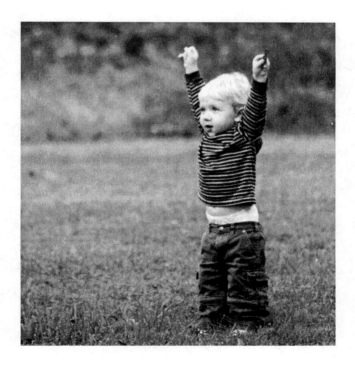

[xxiii] Hu, F.Z. et al. (2000). Mapping of a gene for severe pediatric gastroesophageal reflux to chromosome 13q14. The Journal of the American Medical Association, 284, 325-334.

[xxiv] Reflux Digest. (Spring/Summer 2001. V 5, N 1). Eating problems and reflux-part II, home intervention. p. 11.

[xxv] Reflux Digest. (Summer, 2002. V 6, N 1). Interview with Bill Sears, MD. p. 4.

BEN UPDATE

Just an update on Ben . . . he continues to have good weeks and bad weeks, but is thriving! Food and medicine intolerances remain a big obstacle for us. We have decided to postpone any surgery for the time being and treat his reflux with diet and medication.

We try to keep the real difficulties in mind, and take extra care of ourselves. Without a doubt, this is the hardest thing that we have ever gone through.

Sleep has become our #1 priority. We are still waiting for the time that we sleep through the night, and are usually up anywhere from two to 15 times per night. When we have a few extra minutes or a babysitter we go nap.

We continue to spend a great deal of money on special formula and medications and numerous doctor appointments, but we are trying to focus on all of our other riches.

We remain grateful for jobs that allow us to take off when needed. Our friend list is certainly much smaller than pre-Ben, but that has actually been one of the best parts of his illness. The friends that are left will be with us forever, not just in fair weather. Probably the best thing going for us though is finally putting together a medical team that understands the complexity of acid reflux.

In trying to find some beauty in all of this, we continue to want to make a difference for families that are suffering. Our hope is to someday to do some clinics and try to get as much information to those that need it as possible.

Hang tough,

Tracy and Mike

THANKS

TRACY THANKS
STEWART BARROLL, NANCY AND ZANE CARTER, JERRY AND KIM
CLABAUGH, BOB DENISON, ED FREEMAN, LAURIE KUESTNER, EDIE
HANSON, JULIA HARDING, KATHLEEN HOEY, JUDY LAPRADE,
BRYAN MATTHEWS, JOHN AND TERRI SCHOLL, MARTY SNIDER,
OUR FAMILIES, LINDA WALLS, BONNIE WARD, PHIL WIGGINS, AND
PAT WINTERS FOR HOLDING ME UP WHEN I OTHERWISE WOULD
HAVE FALLEN DOWN . . . BRIANNE BRYNELSON, ANNA GERMAIN,
PEGGY VOSHELL, GAIL GILCHREST, AND KJ WELCENBACH FOR
HOLDING BEN UP WHEN HE COULDN'T LIE DOWN . . . BETH AN-
DERSON AND JAN BURNS FOR BEING REFLUX GODDESSES . . . SUSAN
BAUER, MARCELLA BOTHWELL, STEPHEN LATIMER, AND JEFF PHIL-
LIPS FOR BELIEVING US RIGHT AWAY . . . BRENDA SCRIBNER FOR BE-
ING A TRUTH-SEEKER, AND RICK WIRTZ FOR TRYING TO PUT THE
GOOD STUFF BACK IN.

BEN THANKS
ALL OF HIS RELATIVES FOR THEIR FIGHTING SPIRIT, AND SUSAN
BAUER; MARCELLA BOTHWELL; MARK LANGFITT; STEPHEN
LATIMER; JEFF PHILLIPS; RICK WIRTZ; AND DOLAN, TRISH AND THE
GANG AT EDWARDS PHARMACY; ALL FOR BEING A WONDERFUL
MEDICAL TEAM. HE ALSO THANKS HIS BIG BROTHER FOR CARING
FOR AND LOVING HIM UNCONDITIONALLY.

MIKE THANKS
EACH AND EVERY ONE OF THOSE FOLKS MENTIONED ABOVE. ADDI-
TIONALLY, I WANT TO THANK ALL OF MY WORK-MATES, ESPECIALLY
MY ASSISTANT COACHES OF BRI, CAREN, CHRIS, AND PAT, AND

ALSO JOHN WAGNER, FOR CARRYING THE LOAD WHEN I COULD NOT, AND MY BOSS FOR BEING THE BEST IN THE BUSINESS. MY ATHLETES WERE GREAT—THANKS FOR HELPING AND UNDERSTANDING. JOHN CUNNINGHAM, SAM DAVENPORT, STEW BARROLL AND MARTY SNIDER—YOU WILL NEVER KNOW HOW MUCH OF A DIFFERENCE YOU MADE. DANE ARNOLD—WELL DONE!

FROM ALL OF US A SPECIAL WARM THANKS TO OUR BOOK PRODUCTION TEAM, ESPECIALLY OUR BOOK REVIEWERS (BETH ANDERSON, DON AND MARIANNE BATES, SUSAN BAUER, MARCELLA BOTHWELL, JAN BURNS, ED FRIEMAN, TAMERA GASIOR, NICK KOVIJANIC, DEBBIE PALASKI, JEFFREY PHILLIPS, MACERANA ROSE, BARB SAUER, PATRICIA WINTERS); TO OUR EDITOR, ROBYN ALVAREZ; AND TO OUR COVER DESIGNER, ZANE CARTER.

AND WHO EVER REALLY DID INVENT YOGA, THANKS GREATLY!

INDEX

healthy
  definition, 113
  suggestion to stay, 114
How to Get the Most from
  This Book, 21
How to Read a Book, 90

J
job
  it may suffer, 31

K
Kabat-Zinn, Jon, 128

L
lawyers, 67, 119
LES (lower esophageal
  sphincter), 11

M
medical advice, 18
medical community
  working for you, 61
medical literature, 56, 92
medical recommendations,
  18
medical team
  respect for parents, 73
  respect for them, 73
medical therapist, 33
medications, 14, 28, 30, 48,
  55, 57, 62, 74, 81, 89,

111, 118, 119, 120,125,
  126
  adverse effects, 55
money
  be prepared to spend it,
  117
MSBP. *See* Munchausen
  Syndrome by Proxy
Munchausen Syndrome by
  Proxy, 76

O
online health resources, 83
Our Bodies, Ourselves, 83

P
PAGER, 16, 25, 28, 33, 37,
  46, 65, 75, 80, 82, 103
pain
  baby's, 39
parent
  advocating for your
  baby, 69
  affect of care-giving,
  105
  back pain, 26
  be adaptable, 70
  being supported, 76
  gut check, 77
  improving yourself, 69
  letting go, 70
  quality of life, better, 77
  reducing stress level, 81

Comments Please

How did you like this book? Was it helpful? Want to tell others about it? We're looking for endorsements and testimonials. If you have any you would like to share, let us know. Your help is greatly appreciated. Endorsements usually appear in the following year's edition.

Just fill out the info below, and send off to:

SportWork
Main Street
PO Box 102
Church Hill, MD 21623
(410) 556-6030 (p/f)
tdavenport2@washcoll.edu

Name:		
Address:		
City:	State	Zip:
E-mail:		
Comments:		

Information Update Form

Your feedback is very important to help make this book a better product. If you have information you would like to share, or notice areas of this book that can be improved, let us know.

Just fill out the info below, and send off to:

> SportWork
> PO Box 102
> Main Street
> Church Hill, MD 21623
> (410) 556-6030 (p/f)
> tdavenport2@washcoll.edu

Your help is greatly appreciated. Corrections to the text usually appear in the following year's edition.

Name:		
Address:		
City:	State	Zip:
E-mail:		
Comments:		

Making Life Better —

Quick Order Form

STEP 1: Grab a pen/pencil; **STEP 2:** Complete all information below; **STEP 3:** Mail this form and payment (check / purchase order) to: *SportWork, Main Street, PO Box 192, Church Hill, MD 21623.* (Orders may also be placed at www.makinglifebetter.org.)

Shipping Information

Name:		
Organization:		
Address:		
Address:		
City:	State:	Zip:
Phone:	E-mail:	

Ordering Information

Making Life Better for a Baby With Acid Reflux

	Quantity	*Price*	*Total*
	_____ .	@ $16.95	_____
		Quantity Discount (see below)	_____
		Shipping (free within US, others contact us at 410-556-6030)	_____
		Tax (5% for MD residents)	_____
		Total (prepayment required, pay by credit card at Website)	_____

Discounts:
3–11 books: 20% off retail price
12–36 books: 40% off retail price
37 books and up: 55% off retail price